The Body Clock Diet
24 ways in 24 hours to achieve your ideal weight

Maria Cross

CrossWords Publishing

Published by CrossWords
January 2016
© Maria Cross

Cover design: Peter Cross
Layout: Richard Miller www.richardqmiller.com
Author photo: © Albane Photography

The guidance in this book is for information only and not intended, and should not be seen as, a substitute for medical advice. Always consult a medical practitioner. Use of the information in this book is entirely at the reader's discretion and risk; the author cannot be held responsible for any loss, claim or damage arising out of the use, or misuse, of the suggestions made in this book.

ISBN 978-0-9934760-0-6

The Body Clock Diet

(24) ways in 24 hours to achieve your ideal weight

INTRODUCTION

This is probably not the first time you have set your mind to losing weight, and not the first book you have acquired, with that goal in mind. My aim is to make it the last.

What I offer here is a clear and concise guide to everything that is known about how the body gains and loses weight. This information is presented in twenty-four straightforward sections. Knowledge is power, and in this case knowledge of human metabolism, which has evolved over millions of years to function as it does today, will give you the power to attain your ideal weight as quickly and painlessly as possible.

Weight is a complex issue. Just as there is no single food that will make you fat, there is no single dietary strategy that will instantly make you slim. To focus on one approach – calorie-counting, carbohydrate restriction, fasting or juicing, for example – may help in the short term, but is unlikely to prove sustainable in the long term. What you need, to achieve permanent success, is an approach that embraces the best of all worlds. That is what I present here: the ultimate weight loss toolkit. *The Body Clock Diet* is no one-trick pony; it is a multi-strategy approach, whereby the total effect is greater than the sum of each individual strategy. It is pure weight loss wisdom that works powerfully and effectively to create a slimmer, healthier you.

The Body Clock Diet will transform how you look and how you feel, without making your life a misery. Evolution has programmed your body to metabolise, burn and store food the way it does, and you cannot fight biology. But then, your body was never the enemy; this diet will show you how to work with your metabolism, not against it.

There's something funny going on

The human body houses a finely tuned biochemical clock and once you understand the fundamentals of how this clock works, you will realise that dieting is not only unnecessary, it can lead to even greater weight gain. I've been in this nutrition business for over twenty years, and in all that time I've never met anyone who wanted to be overweight. Yet so many people are, *precisely* because they keep attempting to do what they have been instructed to do: eat less, move more. Why can't you do that?

Dieting can be exhausting as well as futile. It can leave you physically and emotionally drained. Never has such poor advice had such terrible consequences, in terms of health and weight, as you shall see.

If there's one thing that unites humanity across the globe, despite our diversity and our differences, it's fat. We are all fattening at a similar rate, marching in unison towards ever greater fatness. So, if we assume – and I think we can – that very few people are actually happy about this, is it really possible that there has been an exponential rise in people, worldwide, who are simply too lazy to get off their lard-arses to do something about it?

The truth is that in terms of energy we are eating fewer calories now than in the past. The devil, as ever, lies in the detail: we may eat less, but we eat worse. The most recent national diet and nutrition survey, published in 2014, revealed that only 30 per cent of adults meet the five-a-day fruit and vegetable recommendation, and most people eat 'well below' the recommended amount of oily fish.

Tellingly, cereals and cereal products were the 'main contributor to energy intake in all groups', while overall mean fat intake was 'in line with recommendations'. In other words, people are eating a high carbohydrate, low fat diet, just as they have been instructed to do. On average, men aged 19-64 consume 2,111 calories each day, and women 1,613 calories, both figures well below the guidelines – 2,500 calories a day for men, 2,000 for women. Even allowing for under-reporting, which surely we must, it doesn't appear that Mr and Mrs Average are overeating. Yet 26 per cent of men and nearly 24 per cent of women in England are classified as obese. These revelations are seamed with clues to the obesity epidemic.

The more cynically minded might suggest that the strange paradox of eating less but weighing more may be explained by our sedentary lifestyles. Perhaps we are just lazier than ever, slouching on the couch and doing no exercise. However, as you shall see in part six, exercise has surprisingly *little* direct effect on weight, despite its numerous health benefits. Its effects are more *indirect*, when combined with the right diet.

I'm a nutritionist first and foremost. I concern myself with all aspects of health, not just weight issues, but it is evident that obesity and chronic illness such as heart disease, cancer and type 2 diabetes are inextricably linked - to each other, and to our modern diets. The human genome has simply not had time to adapt to our crazy, alien way of eating, if ever it could. Today, we are like a displaced people, living in the wrong time zone, eating the wrong foods and getting the wrong diseases. There is a serious mismatch between what our bodies need and what we give them, so there are bound to be consequences.

Following *The Body Clock Diet* is not just about eating the right foods and avoiding the wrong ones. It's about eating in harmony with your endocrine system and internal body clock. It is an approach that stimulates the hormones that tell you when you are full, and allays those that signal hunger to the brain. It encourages metabolism and favours fat burning over fat accumulation. It eliminates cravings and engenders a healthy attitude to food. In short, *The Body Clock Diet* will guide you towards eating habits that are in tune with your genetic heritage.

In this book I refer to standard measurements of overweight and obesity, even though I personally set little store by them. The body mass index (BMI) is the most common measurement. It is a crude tool, as it does not differentiate between muscle and fat mass. However as a rough guide it is useful, and requires nothing more than a calculator. You calculate your BMI by dividing your weight in kilograms by your height in metres squared. If you check on-line you will find a slew of sites that calculate your BMI for you, once you input your personal data.

BMI

Below 18.5	underweight
18.5 - 24.9	healthy weight
25.0 - 29.9	overweight
30.0 - 30.9	obese
40 plus	morbidly obese

Following *The Body Clock Diet* will bring you to your ideal weight, and along the way you will gain extra bonuses such as improved energy and vitality. You can also expect to reduce your chances of developing chronic illness, such as diabetes and cardiovascular disease. But right now your priority is to lose that unwanted fat and exude loveliness and confidence. Come with me.

The Body Clock Diet

Part One

LET'S START BY GETTING THIS OUT OF THE WAY

The ancient prescription of Hippocrates (400 BC) that the obese should eat less and exercise more continues nowadays to be a widespread approach for weight management despite its well-documented failures. (Dulloo *et al* 2012)

 Never count calories

The first step on your journey is simple and requires very little effort, just commitment. All you have to do is accept that the calorific value of a food item is of absolutely no interest to you. Should you ever find yourself backsliding, covertly performing mental arithmetic at the table, take a deep breath and reread this first part. From here on in you commit to never, ever, counting the calories contained within the food on your plate. It's not natural, it's not helpful and it's not effective.

Don't be too hard on yourselves, you regressors: counting calories is what you have been instructed to do, and what you have done, for longer than you care to remember, to little or no effect. Or rather, to great effect — at first. You reduce your calorie intake substantially, and consequently lose weight. Marvellous! You're hungry, pretty much all the time, but the system's working and you've got the willpower. But soon enough your weight reaches that inevitable plateau. What's more, your hunger is now raging, gnawing at both your stomach and your resolve. Your metabolism has slowed down, your weight loss has flatlined and even eating 'normally' results in weight gain and that creeping sense of despair; you can see what's coming. One emotional trigger, one unkind word, and your willpower crumbles like the cake flashing before your eyes.

The drive to eat when hungry is incredibly powerful. If you restrict calorie intake your body senses the deficit and switches gear. Like a highly trained elite force, a squad of hormones swings into action, and its brief is two-fold: torment you with hunger until your resolve disintegrates, and put the brakes on your metabolism to ensure that you do not burn precious resources.

You really must get off this treadmill.

Over thirty years ago a book was published called *Dieting Makes You Fat* (Cannon & Einzig). Since then, there has been a raft of studies upholding the premise of that book, but that hasn't stopped the experts from urging you to keep doing the same thing, in the hope of getting different results.

Truth is frequently at variance with perception. The world appears flat and still; it is round and spinning. Matter appears mainly solid and inert; it is mainly space and vibrating energy. You eat less, therefore you should weigh less. Fooled again: eat less and you will ultimately weigh more. The strange phenomenon of gaining weight through dieting was first observed in 1945 in what has become a classic study – the Minnesota Starvation Experiment. The aim of this study was to gain insight into the physical and psychological effects of food restriction in starved, war-weary civilians in Europe.

Thirty-six men were put on a diet providing approximately 1,560 calories a day for a period of six months, after first completing a twelve-week control phase during which they were allowed 3,200 calories a day. Participation in the trial was offered to conscientious objectors to the war as an alternative to military service, and although over 400 men volunteered, only those who were deemed to have the mental and physical capacity to see through the experiment were selected. If you consider that the recommended daily intake for men is 2,500 calories you'd be forgiven for thinking that these volunteers were hardly starved. Quite a cushy alternative to going to war, you might think.

It wasn't quite so cushy, as it turned out. During the six-month calorie restriction period, the volunteers lost a quarter of their body weight. They became emaciated and suffered numerous physical and psychological effects, including swelling of the lower limbs, muscle wasting, weakness, apathy, depression and inability to focus. They complained of being cold all the time. They became self-absorbed and anti-social, lost their sense of humour and grew obsessed with food and eating. Nearly 20 per cent showed 'severe character neurosis', with two of the participants becoming borderline psychotic.

Before you go thinking: Hey! That's a small price to pay for all that weight loss, be aware that the metabolic rate of these men decreased by 40 per cent. As a consequence, the pace of weight loss eventually ground to a halt and they were permanently exhausted. Dieting had driven them crazy with hunger, had altered their personalities and left them exhausted. The six-month dieting period was followed by a twelve-week gradual recovery phase, and then an eight-week 'eat all you want' phase. This last step in the experiment must have felt like ascension into food heaven to those poor wretches, but cruelly it turned out to be a descent into a lower circle of hell, with some of the men describing this phase as even more torturous than the calorie restriction period. They could not stop eating, but still felt hungry all the time. They ate almost continuously - over 5,000 and sometimes as many as 10,000 calories per day - and consequently gained weight. This weight was in the form of fat, not muscle, and most of the men completed the trial weighing 10 per cent more than they did at the beginning.

The Minnesota Starvation Experiment was a brutal yet elegant demonstration of the powerful biological system that is activated once you reduce your calorie intake. It's what your body does when it senses a food shortage, in an effort to retain energy stores. In other words, it's what happens when you go on a diet. Since the Minnesota experiment was published, numerous other studies have also concluded that dieting is associated with long term weight gain, and that the more attempts made to lose weight, the greater the chances of gaining it. This phenomenon has even been given a name: fat overshooting. Charming, but nevertheless.

Fat overshooting is considered a paradox, but there's nothing paradoxical about the body's metabolism, designed through evolution to enhance our chances of survival. The body is equipped with defensive reactions to negative energy balance and will restore any weight lost, *beyond the point of weight restoration*. In other words, you will regain the weight that you lost, and then some.

The traditional calorie reduction diet is based on the first law of thermodynamics, a law which applies beautifully to internal combustion engines, but not so much to the human body. According to this law, obesity is a disorder of energy imbalance. When calories-in exceed calories-out, there is an energy surplus which will be stored as fat. The simplicity of this theory is so intuitively appealing that it has endured, and continues to endure, despite all the evidence to the contrary. Calories exist and they do matter, but how much food you eat and how the body uses it is contingent upon much more than its calorific value. The human body, unlike a combustion engine, is a complex living organism, driven by ancient survival mechanisms involving hormones and enzymes that govern every aspect of appetite and metabolism. They effectively decide whether you store or burn fat, and whether your brain's reward centres are satisfied with what you have eaten or instead issue overwhelming demands for you to keep going.

Anyone who studies the science of weight and metabolism surely knows all this, so it is puzzling that this information is ignored by those invested with the task of providing the best available advice on the subject. The NHS Choices website, developed by dietitians from the British Dietetic Association, remains firmly entrenched in the doctrine of calorie counting (and eating plenty of carbohydrates and low fat products – more later on why this is such a bad idea). You are advised that *to lose weight, you need to eat and drink fewer calories than you use each day*. Men are advised to consume no more than 1,900kcal a day and women 1,400kcal. (Minnesota Starvation Experiment, anyone?) The NHS even helpfully provides details of on-line calorie counters. If you go over the prescribed amount one day, you have to reduce your intake proportionately over the following days. It's a system that has never worked and is guaranteed to ultimately fail. Good luck with that.

Finally, as you may have already learned from experience, calorie restriction is psychologically and emotionally stressful and can result in depression, anxiety and irritability. It can also create an unhealthy, obsessive relationship with food. You will read about how stress can contribute to fat gain in part six.

Calories matter, in that the body has to do something with the energy you consume. But not all calories are created equally. Some, depending on their source, will be stored immediately as fat and others will be burned for energy. Some will blunt your appetite and others will stimulate it. All this will become clear as you progress through this book. As you do so, remain mindful that your focus is fat loss – not muscle, organ tissue, bone or fluids. Just fat. And remember too that there is a world of difference between the fat you eat and the fat you want to burn – the fat stored in your adipose tissue. It's this adipose tissue that you are going to demolish.

Now that you know what you are *not* going to do, it is time to move on to the practicalities of what you are going to do, in order to reduce your fat stores and achieve your ideal weight. You are not going to eat less; you are going to eat smart.

Takeaway

- Calorie restriction results in a reduction in metabolic rate
- A calorie restricted diet ultimately results in weight gain
- The human body has evolved hormonal systems which prevent the breakdown of fat when food is scarce
- Calorie restriction creates stress and may lead to an unhealthy obsession with food

Part Two

WAKEY WAKEY! TIME TO START YOUR PRE-BREAKFAST ROUTINE

Other than breast milk, the only drink anyone needs is water.
Everything else... is surplus to human requirements, but a life
with nothing else to drink might be a tad dull. (Cross 2013)

(2) Drink the right kind of tea

Most people start the day with a hot drink, and this common ritual offers an early opportunity to set your body to weight loss mode.

Tea, specifically green tea, may actually aid weight loss, surprisingly enough. It sounds like one of those marketing myths put about by the purveyors of would-be wonder products, but research has in fact revealed that green tea can help reduce fat mass and waist circumference in overweight and obese people. This effect is achieved through improved metabolic rate and fat oxidation, as observed in a number of studies.

Green tea has been highlighted more than once as a potential weight loss aid. There has been quite a bit of research, and (after discarding a large number of questionable trials) a review of eleven robust studies found that certain chemicals in green tea – catechins – can significantly help decrease body weight, and keep it off. Common sense is required here: throwing back mugs of tea all day long is not likely to have much effect on its own, but when combined with the other dietary strategies outlined in this book, green tea consumption can contribute to the efficiency and speed at which the weight drops off.

Green tea is something of an acquired taste. It is quite bitter, unless you drink it fairly weak, in which case it is light and refreshing. I talk from experience here – I make a pot with just one teaspoon and find that hits the spot perfectly. (You may prefer to use a teabag, but I'm a purist when it comes to tea and prefer loose leaf.) No milk is required and as you shall see further on, the less milk you drink the better.

If you really are loath to give up your normal brew, that's fine. Black tea also contains catechins, though to a much lesser extent than green tea.

(3) **Get your coffee kicks**

Coffee is also an effective weight loss tool, albeit via a more indirect route than tea. Caffeine has been found, in many studies ongoing since the 1960s, to reduce the risk of developing type 2 diabetes. This effect appears to be dose-dependent: the more coffee consumed, the lower the risk. It is probably for this reason that it helps prevent fat gain; you will see in part three how weight gain and diabetes are strongly linked, and that by reducing the risk of diabetes you simultaneously reduce the risk of gaining weight.

Exercise caution with milk. A small splash two or three times a day is fine, but lay off the lattes and the cappuccinos for reasons that will become apparent in part four.

In addition to tea and/or coffee, drink plenty of water throughout the morning. You have been processing digested food all night, and as all metabolic activity requires water you need to replenish supplies for the day that lies ahead. Tea and coffee may also be drunk at other times of the day.

Jettison the juicer

If you habitually start the day with a fruit juice, kick this habit into touch now.

Fruit is marvellous, and certainly has a place on this programme. Fruit juice, on the other hand, is less than marvellous and has no place. Fruit is naturally high in fibre, and as a whole food offers plenty of nutrition with relatively little fruit sugar (which might surprise you). Strip that fruit of its fibre content and you are left with water and concentrated fruit sugar.

High fructose (fruit sugar) is of particular concern to you, because you are attempting to lose fat, and fat is what you get from drinking fruit juices. The fructose found in fruit juice is concentrated, and because the body has no use for this amount of sugar, the liver converts it into fat so that it can be put into storage. Excess fructose can also lead to the formation of damaged proteins called advanced glycation end products. These damaged proteins accumulate along artery walls and contribute to plaque formation, which can result in thrombosis. So not only does fructose contribute to weight gain, it doesn't do your arteries or life expectancy any good either.

Fructose is selective about where it fattens you, favouring the accumulation of abdominal and ectopic fat over other areas. Ectopic fat is fat that accumulates in areas where it wouldn't normally: around the heart, the liver or in muscles. It is therefore dangerous as well as undesirable.

There's more. Fructose consumption reduces circulating leptin. Leptin is a hormone, made in adipose tissue (your fat store), which signals to the brain that fat cells are adequately filled, so acts as an appetite suppressant. Lower your leptin and you will automatically increase your appetite. So fruit juice not only does nothing to fill you up, it actually makes you more hungry.

Takeaway

- Green tea and coffee consumption can help stimulate weight loss
- Fructose contributes to the development of arterial plaques and fat around organs such as the heart
- Fruit juice consumption encourages fat gain and increases hunger

---

Part Three

YOUR FIRST MEAL

From a public health perspective, redistribution of daily energy intake, so that a larger percentage is consumed at breakfast and a lower percentage is consumed over the rest of the day, may help to reduce weight gain in middle-aged adults. (Purslow *et al* 2008)

(5) Eat when you're ready

You've slept well and had a nice cup of tea or coffee; now it's time to start the day. This does not mean eating as soon as you have come round.

Most people do not actually feel like eating first thing in the morning, but think they should because they have been told for as long as they can remember that breakfast is the most important meal of the day. Without breakfast to provide energy for the day ahead they risk collapsing into a feeble heap. It is ironic that, at the one time of day when you really don't feel like it, you are told that you must eat something.

There is a reason why most people have little or no appetite when they wake up: the human body clock and the production of cortisol. Cortisol is an adrenal hormone produced cyclically: levels start to rise between 3am and 6am, and within thirty to forty minutes after waking most people experience a two- to three-fold surge in circulating cortisol. With cortisol comes energy, in what is termed the 'awakening cortisol response'. This surge in cortisol, and mobilisation of energy reserves, explains why most of us do not wake up with a ravenous appetite and why so many people manage a pre-breakfast workout in the gym without passing out, or perhaps go for a brisk walk before breakfast, in order to work up an appetite.

That is not to say that metabolic disturbances do not occur: people with diabetes and the metabolic syndrome (more of this later) are more likely to suffer from low energy in the morning and may need to eat soon after waking. If you are someone who has habitually eaten a high carbohydrate diet, you may also have a mild blood sugar imbalance that means that you cannot fast for prolonged periods without feeling light-headed, a bit shaky, irritable and unable to concentrate.

It is important therefore that you have a good appetite before you eat. If you are not hungry, it's because you still have fuel in your blood so anything you eat will be surplus to requirements and end up in storage.

Better late than never

Do not worry if this means having a late breakfast. Breakfast does matter, because a raft of studies have concluded that skipping this meal can lead to weight gain. You may find this to be counter-intuitive; surely by eating less you should weigh less. Not so: a large breakfast is satisfying, and studies have found that you are more likely to eat larger quantities later in the day if you skip this meal, or do not eat enough. Don't be afraid to eat a big breakfast, because the more food you consume earlier in the day, the more your fat burning efficiency at night. Researchers of one particular study of over 6,700 adults aged 40-75 found that the more total daily calories the participants consumed at breakfast, compared to any other meal, the more likely they were to have a lower body mass index compared to people who consumed more of their total calories as the evening meal. The authors of the study concluded that redistributing daily energy intake - consuming more in the morning and less later in the day - may help reduce weight gain.

The important thing is to eat when hungry (this may be an hour or two, or even more, after waking) and as we shall now see, to make it a protein based meal.

(6) Control your insulin

It is said that you can have too much of a good thing, and never a truer word was said when it comes to the hormone insulin. Without it you're either dead or diabetic, but with too much you could find yourself fat and sick. Keeping circulating levels tightly under control is central to both weight loss and good health.

Insulin is a hormone released by the pancreas when food is eaten, mainly in response to glucose in the blood. Glucose is derived from the carbohydrate that you eat. Carbohydrates include cereals and other starchy foods. In order to understand (and accept) why you will not be consuming cereals, muffins, toast and the like for breakfast you need to understand the role of the hormone insulin, and to know where you're coming from.

Insulin performs quite a few tasks, but in terms of weight management it has three major roles, as explained below.

First, insulin regulates blood sugar. Eat carbohydrates

and your digestive system will get to work on them, breaking them down into smaller molecules of glucose and then transporting those molecules through the gut lining and into the bloodstream. That is how sugar enters your blood. This sugar – glucose - needs to be tightly regulated. Too much and you are in potential danger. You have only (or should have only) around a teaspoon of sugar coursing through your blood vessels at any given time. More than that and you could be in trouble, which is where insulin comes in. It takes excess glucose and sends it off for storage in your muscles and liver, where it becomes known as glycogen. When these depositories are full – and they have limited storage capacity – off goes that surplus glucose to your adipose tissue. It has now become fat.

The second main role of insulin therefore concerns fat storage. You only have room for around 2,000 calories in your muscles and liver, but the storage capacity of your adipose tissue is prodigious and all too visible. Insulin regulates an enzyme called lipoprotein lipase (LPL) whose job it is to pull fat from blood into either muscle or adipose tissue. The more carbohydrate you consume, the more insulin you secrete, and the more insulin you secrete, the more active LPL becomes on fat cells. Voilà – you've just got fatter. Not by eating fat, but by eating carbohydrate.

The third main role of insulin is to block the flow of fat out of adipose tissue if glucose levels remain high. Fat stays locked away, every exit blocked by zealous insulin guards. With your fat secured firmly under lock and key, you crave more carbohydrates as fuel. And so the cycle continues.

From evolution to revolution

Your body clock is calibrated precisely as it was when you first emerged as a fully fledged *Homo sapiens* in equatorial Africa and packed your tools to go a-hunting. That was roughly two hundred thousand years ago.

The human body evolved on a diet of mainly meat, offal, fish, bone marrow, fruit and other wild plant foods. You would have also helped yourself to nuts and seeds when available, depending on where you and yours settled after leaving equatorial east Africa, our original homeland. Those of you whose ancestors headed towards the Arctic tundra (why?) would have relied almost exclusively on fish, seal meat and blubber. Others who chose to settle in more temperate zones would have eaten more plant foods. When they got lucky, they enjoyed a sweet treat, honey. Availability was seasonal and obtaining it fraught with danger, so honey was not something to be enjoyed on a daily basis. Your ancestors very much liked this rare treat though, an omen perhaps of diets to come.

For reasons that remain elusive we took it upon ourselves, a mere 11,000 years ago, to revolutionise the way we eat and live. This global revolution created such a seismic shift in lifestyle that it changed forever the meaning of being human. We exchanged survival skills and a sense of connectedness to the natural environment for society, science, politics and religion. With this new lifestyle came a profound change in diet. We switched from hunter-gathering to cultivating cereal grasses. It cost us: analyses of skeletal remains have revealed that the impact of this nutrition transition was staggering, in terms of health.

Weaker bone density, lower stature, poor dental health, anaemia and greater susceptibility to infection were the price these early agriculturalists of the neolithic era paid for their change in diet.

Even so, these changes were of nothing compared to what was to come, thousands of years further down the time-line: the Industrial Revolution and subsequent birth of the junk food industry. Industrialisation ushered in an era of food processing on a massive, hitherto unknown scale. It was as if we'd all moved to another planet serving a different menu.

As we left the fields for the towns, we also left the responsibility for providing our food to the new captains of industry. We developed a taste for their novel, mass-produced, highly refined cereals, and once sugar was added to the equation, we were addicted. White bread, white rice, sugary breakfast cereals, cakes, biscuits… they were posh, they were white, they were trash.

It was during this wave of industrial creativity that we were to truly embrace technologies that made us fat as well as sick. Industry was on a high, seeking out ever more innovative ways to provide food in bulk for expanding urban populations and their waistlines. We didn't just eat cereal grains – we refined them too, removing the germ and bran and leaving just pure white flour that could be stored for lengthy periods without spoiling. Then we found ingenious ways of adding sugar to these refined cereal grains and calling it a great breakfast, or even an energy snack. These foods are not the natural order of things, and neither is fatness, but together they have merged to become the norm. The phenomenal changes to the human diet that have taken place since the Industrial Revolution – or indeed the beginning of agriculture - have been far too rapid for adaptation by the human genome.

This is where insulin comes in...

Foods especially high in carbohydrate include bread, potatoes, rice, pasta, corn... in other words those starches that are newcomers to the human diet. A diet of unlimited, novel carbohydrates puts immense pressure on the pancreas to keep pumping out insulin on a level it was not designed for. There have to be consequences, as indeed there are.

Keep producing large quantities of insulin and you risk becoming immune to it. Being immune to insulin is called insulin resistance. Insulin resistance is a modern phenomenon, and is the impetus behind what are frequently referred to as 'diseases of civilisation': obesity, cancer, type 2 diabetes, hypertension and cardiovascular disease. Insulin resistance is a blood sugar disorder whereby either the liver or muscles no longer respond adequately to insulin in the blood, or the pancreas is no longer able to keep producing sufficient insulin to deal with the never-ending glucose. If the liver and muscles do not respond to all this circulating insulin, glucose in the blood remains high. It has to go somewhere, however, and fat cells are only too happy to take up the slack, with the abdomen being the most favoured region. That is why people with insulin resistance tend to have fat bellies. Insulin resistance is caused by a relentless intake of refined carbohydrates and sugar that eventually takes its toll. It's not that your body is defective when it comes to coping with your diet; your diet is defective and ill-suited to the genetic design of your body.

Metabolic mayhem

If you have insulin resistance (and plenty of people do) and you keep up this sort of diet for long enough, there is every chance you'll end up not only fat but with something called the metabolic syndrome. The metabolic syndrome is a cluster of symptoms (obesity, high blood pressure, high blood fats, high blood sugar) that increase your risk of developing heart disease, stroke, type 2 diabetes and even dementia, which is why researchers now frequently refer to Alzheimer's as type 3 diabetes. The brain is highly sensitive to glucose, and high levels of insulin can interfere with cognitive function, including memory and concentration. Research suggests that more than 80 per cent of Alzheimer's patients have either type 2 diabetes or abnormal blood glucose levels. That itself is good enough reason to keep insulin levels under control. Being overweight is a classic symptom of the metabolic syndrome, so losing weight is a proactive route to good health.

You are no different from your lean, super-fit forebears; your body has absolutely no requirement for sugar and starchy carbohydrates. We have been told so often that bread, rice, potatoes *et al* are essential staples that we have come to accept this baseless dogma. Don't believe the hype – even the wholegrain varieties of these starches, such as wholemeal bread, contain unremarkable levels of nutrients compared to other foods.

Fruits and vegetables also contain carbohydrates but these are in another, perfectly acceptable league, as I shall later explain.

Index linked

What these foods do have is a high glycaemic index. The glycaemic index is a system that measures the rate at which the glucose component of a food item enters the blood and raises blood sugar levels, and therefore insulin, on a score of 0-100. A low GI is a score of 55 or less, a medium GI is 56-69 and a high GI score is 70 or over.

Cereals and grains - including 'whole' grains - have shockingly high GIs to match their low nutrient values. Wholemeal bread, for example, has a GI of 69 – only one point less than white bread. Wholegrain brown rice, the flagship food of every be-sandalled healthnik, notches up a not-so-healthy 76, and in its refined white form scores a shameful 90, which is almost like eating pure glucose.

The glycaemic index of some starchy carbohydrates

Croissant	67
Weetabix	69
Wholemeal bread	69
Chips	75
Brown rice	76
Rice cakes	82
Popcorn	85
White rice	90

All these starchy carbohydrates simply have to go. This rule also applies to beans and lentils and vegetables such as swede and celeriac. Ordinarily, I would recommend these plant foods, as they are nutritious and high in fibre. Indeed, they feature on the maintenance programme, as outlined in part seven. However, as your goal is to lose fat - and I'm assuming you want to do so as fast as it is feasible and healthy to do so - the fewer starchy carbohydrates you eat the better, in order for your body to switch from burning glucose to burning stored fat.

> See the tables in appendix one for details of which carbohydrates you should avoid, and which are acceptable to eat, when following *The Body Clock Diet*.

Clearly it is essential that you limit your insulin production, in order to burn your adipose tissue. No other hormone will fatten you quite as efficiently as insulin; it drives the accumulation of body fat and prevents it from being oxidised for energy. To actively minimise insulin secretion you need to embark on a low carbohydrate way of eating. This is precisely the way your lean but well-nourished hunter-gatherer ancestors ate.

There is no official consensus on what constitutes a low carbohydrate diet. Having said that, daily consumption of fewer than 50 grams of carbohydrate is generally accepted to be low. There is plenty of compelling evidence to show that a low carbohydrate diet is superior to a low fat diet as an effective weight loss measure. We have known this for long enough, but these facts are always slow to make their way from research to common knowledge. Here's just one example, published in *Annals of Internal Medicine* in 2004: 120 overweight volunteers followed either a low carbohydrate diet or a low fat, low cholesterol, low calorie diet. Participants in both groups carried out exercise and attended group meetings. At 24 weeks, average weight loss was considerably greater in the low carbohydrate group – 9.4 kilos, as opposed to 4.8 kilos in the low fat group. Furthermore, those on the low carbohydrate diet had greater reductions in blood fat levels and higher levels of HDL cholesterol, outcomes that are considered protective of heart health. Tellingly, many more of the low carbohydrate group than the low fat group were able to complete the study (76 per cent versus 57 per cent).

From reading the research it becomes apparent that this sort of result is the rule rather than the exception, and that the lower the intake of energy from carbohydrate, the greater the weight loss. A low carbohydrate diet works because it reduces insulin secretion and stimulates the mobilisation of fat from storage. It also leads to a reduction in appetite – a welcome phenomenon that has been observed in numerous studies.

From now on, you will be eating a satisfying, protein-based breakfast. Although the same also goes for lunch and dinner, it is especially important that you eat a high protein (and low carbohydrate) breakfast, as this will regulate your appetite for the whole day. High protein breakfasts elicit the greatest satiety, reducing the urge to snack, even in the evening, an effect not observed in people consuming a carbohydrate based breakfast. You will also have less desire to overeat in the evening, which is crucial to fat burning. In addition to its other fine qualities, a protein based breakfast has been found to reduce daily ghrelin secretion, something that doesn't happen when you eat a cereal based breakfast. Ghrelin is a hormone produced by the stomach that tells your brain you are hungry, and the less of that the better.

Following *The Body Clock Diet* quickly balances blood sugar and increases energy levels. Take out all those unnecessary carbohydrates and prepare to be amazed at how much more energised you feel, especially in the morning. From now on set your body clock to appetite and metabolic control for the rest of the day by consuming no toast, no cereal (not exactly a hardship) and no croissants (ok, a bit). Just good old-fashioned protein: eggs, bacon, sausage, cold meats, cheese, fish. You'll find it satisfying, and you'll feel great too. That's what it is to feel normal, to feel human.

Don't go soft

The day stretches ahead, and perhaps you habitually fuel the post-prandial hours with a soft drink or two. This is another habit that you are going to have to ditch.

It has long been suspected that soft drinks make a hefty contribution to the obesity epidemic. There is strong evidence that sugar-sweetened drinks promote weight gain and obesity in young children, adolescents and adults. You saw earlier how sugar causes a marked rise in insulin, and insulin favours fat accumulation. Sugary drinks are worse than sugary foods, because they have no impact on satiety. You can drink and drink as much as you like, but you will never feel full, despite all that sugar and all those calories. Consequently you will not eat any less. Instead, you will find yourself on the path to insulin resistance and inflammation and anything and everything associated with the metabolic syndrome. I cannot think of anything more pointless than a soft drink.

Fake is futile

So, you're thinking, I can carry on with my soft drinks habit as long as my fix is sugar-free and calorie-free, and only sweetened with artificial chemicals. Wrong! In the past it was always assumed that zero-calorie drinks could make a worthwhile contribution to any weight loss programme. I might point out that you can obtain a similar worthwhile effect by avoiding all soft drinks. In fact you'd be better off, as these artificial sweeteners appear to do more harm than good. When fourteen men with type 2 diabetes were given, at different times, either a high sugar meal, a fructose-based meal, an aspartame-sweetened meal or a high-fat meal, it was expected that the aspartame-sweetened meal would have the lowest impact on insulin release and blood sugar. *'Contrary to all expectations'*, the results revealed that the aspartame meal induced a rise in glucose and insulin levels similar to that of the high sugar meal. In other words, artificial sweeteners have the same effect on blood sugar as real sugar. In mice, consumption of sweeteners has been found to significantly increase body weight, despite no change in food intake. Of mice and men: according to the researchers, these results call into question the effect of these artificial sweeteners on weight loss in humans. Best avoided – stick with your tea and coffee and of course plenty of natural, thirst-quenching water.

Takeaway

- High morning cortisol levels mean you don't have to eat the moment you wake up
- Insulin secretion needs to be kept low, as high insulin encourages the storage of fat and prevents it from being burned
- Research has consistently found a low carbohydrate diet to be more effective than a low fat, low calorie diet
- A low carbohydrate diet reduces the risk of chronic disease such as cardiovascular disease and type 2 diabetes
- A high protein breakfast regulates appetite for the rest of the day
- Soft drinks do not fill you up but instead contribute to weight gain
- Artificial sweeteners are no better than ordinary sugar as they cause a rise in blood sugar and contribute to weight gain

Part Four

FROM NOON TILL NIGHT

*We found that severely obese subjects with a high prevalence
of diabetes and the metabolic syndrome lost more weight in
a six-month period on a carbohydrate-restricted diet than
on a fat- and calorie-restricted diet... Subjects in this group
may have experienced greater satiety on a diet with liberal
proportions of protein and fat.* (Samaha et al 2003)

 ## Don't be a cow

You will be eating three times a day on *The Body Clock Diet*.
Snacking is not necessary; we humans are not grazing
beasts whose every waking moment requires us to have
our snouts to the trough. Snacking is a luxury of the
well-fed world, a world that struggles to recognise when
enough is enough. Following this programme requires that
you refrain from eating between meals. This will give you
time to digest and metabolise your food and start burning
fat stores. Your hunter-gatherer ancestors did not graze
on precious resources just because they were bored or
fed-up. Their high protein, high fat diet ensured that their
appetite was sated whilst they got on with hunting, setting
traps, building shelters and whittling tools.

You don't have the guts

We omnivores are genetically adapted to a high protein,
high fat diet that allows us to spend most of our time

doing things other than eating; herbivorous mammals, on the other hand, have to eat throughout the day. There are two types of herbivore, and through evolution they have developed complex digestive systems to manage the large amount of plant matter they consume. Cellulose in plants is much more difficult to break down than animal tissue, so requires specific systems that can handle the task. The first type of herbivore is the ruminant, which has a complex, four-chambered stomach to facilitate the breakdown of raw plant material. This group includes cattle, goats and deer. The second type of herbivore – the hindgut fermenter – is a bulk feeder with an enlarged caecum and large, complex colon to ferment food, most of which passes through the intestines undigested. This group includes elephants, horses and rabbits. You have neither a four-chambered stomach nor an enlarged colon and caecum; instead, you are equipped with a simple stomach and short colon, features that are characteristic of meat-eating mammals. Whether you like it or not, you are ill-equipped for a raw, vegetarian diet but perfectly equipped for a diet of meat and plant foods.

If you take to grazing - snacking - throughout the day, your fat stores will remain firmly locked away; you will not draw on this reserve if you keep topping up your blood with fuel. Don't panic - because your meals will all be protein and fat based, appetite is something that will build gradually and you will not feel an urgent need to reach for a quick fix. There will be none of that desperate craving associated with plummeting blood sugar levels that you may have experienced back in the day when you regularly feasted on carbohydrates. The idea that you should eat 'little and often' is nonsense and is a quick-fix remedy for the blood-sugar-disrupting effects of a high carbohydrate diet.

Fruit and nut case

There are two compromises regarding the no-snacking rule, and the first applies to the morning period. A total of two pieces of fruit may be consumed in the morning, just before breakfast or lunch. Fruit offers valuable nutrition and the phytochemicals it contains can actively promote weight loss (you'll read about this soon). Some fruits do have a relatively high carbohydrate content, so are best avoided – see appendix one for which fruits to eat and which to avoid on *The Body Clock Diet*. Carbohydrates are metabolised faster in the morning than at any other time of the day; fruit is quickly metabolised and its consumption, especially in the morning, will have no impact on weight. Unlike other sugars, fructose does not cause insulin spikes, so the amount found in fresh fruit is harmless. Dried fruit however is off the menu. Without water, the sugar content soars and concentrated fructose is not a good thing, as you have seen.

The great thing about fruits (and vegetables) is that they are self-limiting. You might eat a piece of fruit and feel satisfied with that; not many people have to fight off cravings for a second, or third. The same goes for vegetables – you know when you've had enough. The same cannot be said for starchy, carbohydrate-based snack foods, as you probably already know.

It's up to you how you do this: either have two pieces of fruit just before breakfast or lunch, or have one piece just before either meal.

The second exception to the snacking rule is this: if dinner is delayed (that is, is to be eaten more than five hours after lunch) or lunch was insubstantial, have a small handful of plain nuts, about half an hour or less before eating. Good choices include Brazils, hazelnuts, macadamias, cashews, pecans and walnuts… all nuts are good, as long as they are not roasted in vegetable oil. These highly nutritious nibbles will allay any hunger and have no impact on weight. They will also ensure you are not tempted to overeat when dinner is ready. Remember, this strategy is applicable only if dinner is delayed or lunch insubstantial. Nuts have virtually no carbohydrate, but plenty of minerals, fat and protein. One mineral they have in spades is magnesium, and magnesium helps calm the nervous system, making evening consumption especially apposite. They are also a surprisingly good source of antioxidants, those naturally occurring chemicals that keep heart disease, cancer and other chronic but common diseases at bay. As well as allaying hunger before dinner, they can also easily be incorporated into meals, especially breakfast or lunch. For those of you who don't like nuts, or are allergic to them, try a handful of olives (in brine, not oil) instead. Olives contain virtually no carbohydrate and are full of fibre and monounsaturated fat – more on this later.

 ## Get your timing right (part 1)

Once you have eaten your low carbohydrate, high protein breakfast, you will eat nothing for at least four hours. When lunchtime comes you will – again – have a quality protein with two portions of cooked vegetables or salad.

> See appendix one for vegetable suggestions and
> appendix two for suggested lunchbox items.

Obviously, any fish or meat that you may have won't be of the bread-crumbed or battered variety, and the same goes for your evening meal. Most vegetables are permitted, but there are a few exceptions, due to their high carbohydrate content – see appendix one. Four hours is about right, but again you need to monitor your appetite: if you have no appetite, it is too soon to eat. The larger your breakfast, the longer you'll find you can wait for lunch.

10 Fan those fat-burning flames

Eating quality protein is your passport to effortless weight loss. By making protein the focus of each meal you can expect to experience a reduction in appetite and an upsurge in energy. By eating more protein not only do you lose weight quickly and painlessly, you gain better musculature. A low carbohydrate, high protein diet positively influences body mass and composition, regardless of the number of calories consumed.

Protein power is no mystery – obesity researchers have long observed that greater protein consumption is one of the most direct routes to weight loss. We have already seen that calorie restriction works in the short term, but in the long term can have disastrous consequences. A higher protein diet works in both the short and the long term and not only keeps your appetite sated, it promotes good health and vitality too.

Proteins form a significant proportion of bone, muscle, skin, organs, glands, hormones, enzymes, antibodies, neurotransmitters, DNA ... around 20 per cent of body mass is protein. Proteins make things that make things happen: they build and repair, they strengthen, metabolise, transport and store.

Animal magic

A protein is a body of amino acids. There are 22 amino acids, nine of which are considered essential. Essential in this case means they must be obtained from the diet; the non-essential amino acids can be synthesised from the essential ones. Foods that contain all nine essential amino acids are referred to as 'complete' or 'quality' proteins. The only foods that contain a complete protein, with a couple of exceptions, are animal-based foods: meat, fish, eggs and dairy. There are few plant exceptions, the main ones being soya beans and quinoa. Soya beans (and soya products such as tofu) are a staple food for many vegetarians and vegans as they offer reasonable levels of protein, though nowhere near as much as meat and fish. However they also contain significant amounts of carbohydrate and omega-6 fatty acids. You will see later on why you do not want omega-6 fatty acids in high amounts if you want to lose weight. Quinoa, which although a seed is treated from a culinary perspective as a cereal grain, also contains all the essential amino acids, but contrary to popular myth is very low in protein overall and is predominantly (over 70 per cent) carbohydrate. Quorn, for those of you who are wondering, does not even qualify as a food, in my book, let alone a protein. There is no such thing growing or living anywhere. It is fabricated in a laboratory from soil mould and in my view embodies all that is heinous about commercial food production. We'll say no more.

The vanishing appetite

As you saw in part one, being hungry much of the time is counterproductive. Reduce your calorie intake and after a while your body will start to break down lean tissue to provide fuel whilst conserving fat stores. Incessant hunger drives you crazy and engenders an unhealthy relationship with food. Every dieter's dream is an appetite so under control that hours can pass without a pang. Your dream has come true, as that is exactly what you can expect on a high protein diet.

That is also precisely the sort of diet that your hunter-gatherer ancestors ate and indeed survived on. Survival meant efficiency, and efficiency meant optimal foraging – energy obtained from food should be greater than the amount of energy expended obtaining that food. Working cooperatively to bring down large prey provided a great deal of energy in the form of protein and fat - enough to satisfy an entire tribe. Spending all day gathering berries and leaves is not going to cut the mustard, in terms of optimal foraging, especially when you are living in the middle of an ice age, have an almost hairless body and spend most of your time exposed to the elements.

Protein is even more filling than fat, despite containing fewer calories per gram. Fat has nine calories per gram, protein four. In studies, a diet consisting of 30 per cent protein has been found to 'markedly' increase satiety, and to lead to a spontaneous reduction in food intake. How does protein do this? The answer is believed to lie in its ability to influence certain hormones that regulate appetite. One of these hormones is ghrelin. Ghrelin is secreted in the stomach and stimulates appetite by acting as a hunger signal to the brain. Therefore, as you'd expect, levels of ghrelin rise during calorie restriction. Interesting experiments have revealed that giving volunteers ghrelin as an infusion increases appetite and voluntary food intake, an effect observed in both obese and lean people. Naturally, you don't want any ghrelin infusions. Quite the contrary; part of your plan is to prevent ghrelin tormenting you all day, and that is precisely what protein does. It suppresses concentrations of this hormone once you have finished eating, and for prolonged periods thereafter. What's more, protein increases levels of two key hormones that work in opposition to ghrelin by suppressing hunger: polypeptide YY (PYY) and cholecystokinin (CCK).

PYY is secreted along the digestive tract; levels increase after eating, and decrease during fasting. CCK is stimulated by both protein and fat, and produces satiety by slowing down the rate at which food passes out of the stomach ('gastric emptying' is the terminology) so you feel fuller for longer. This has been found to have the effect of inhibiting food intake quite markedly. CCK, which also stimulates the release of digestive enzymes by the pancreas, has been the subject of some intense research over the last thirty years because of its influence on the gut-brain pathway. It is found throughout the small intestine and is released after eating. In the same way that giving someone an infusion of ghrelin can increase appetite, administration of CCK has been found to induce the feeling of fullness. Indeed, multiple studies have found that administered CCK suppresses food intake and hunger ratings. You don't need any infusions, as you are not a lab rat – you just have to eat a high protein and fat diet to suppress ghrelin and stimulate plenty of CCK and PYY naturally.

Burn, baby

A high protein diet not only promotes appetite control, it speeds up fat loss. It does this by increasing thermogenesis, your resting metabolic rate. Protein does this better than fat or carbohydrate, all the while preserving lean body mass. The problem with prolonged fasting is that it can cause muscle to be broken down and used for glucose production. This you do not want, because it means you are losing tone, and not burning fat. A large number of studies have confirmed that after eating protein, the body burns fat *at an accelerated rate*. What's more, this effect has been found to be immediate, which is terrific because you want to lose weight in the here and now, not on another time and space continuum. Protein not only favours the retention of lean muscle, it actually improves muscle metabolism. When a group of 130 participants (men and women aged 40-56) were given either a high protein (meat, dairy, eggs and nuts), low carbohydrate diet, or a low protein, high carbohydrate diet (bread, rice, cereals, pasta and potatoes) for four months, those in the high protein group lost 22 per cent more fat mass than the high carbohydrate group. What's more, after twelve months more people (64 per cent compared to 45 per cent) were still following the high protein diet, and had experienced greater improvement in body composition. The protein group experienced 28 per cent greater fat loss, even though these two groups consumed the same number of calories throughout. That is what is known as a result.

Similar results were found in another, smaller study of seventeen obese men aged 20-65 with a BMI of 30 plus, reported in the *American Journal of Clinical Nutrition*. They were recruited to participate in a trial comparing the hunger and appetite responses of either a high protein, low carbohydrate diet or a medium carbohydrate diet. Both diets contained exactly the same number of calories. The participants followed one of the two diets for a period of four weeks before changing over to the other diet. At the end of the trial it was found that they felt significantly less hungry, and therefore chose to eat a lot less (40 per cent fewer calories) when they were on the high protein, low carbohydrate diet. Weight loss was also significantly greater on this diet (6.34 kilos compared to 4.35 kilos on the medium carbohydrate diet).

The best quality proteins are meat, fish, seafood, eggs and cheese. Ensure you eat plenty of fish for the omega-3 fatty acids EPA and DHA which you will soon be reading about. White fish is an excellent source of complete protein, even if it contains little EPA and DHA. Plaice, haddock, sole etc. are very decent proteins and make a welcome occasional change from meat and oily fish.

But is it healthy?

If you balk at the thought of eating a lot of meat from a health perspective, there's no need. The study I mentioned above, where the high protein group lost 28 per cent more body fat than the high carbohydrate group, also found that by the end of the year the protein group were healthier all round – blood tests revealed lower triglycerides (the form of fat in the blood which is considered a health risk) and higher HDL cholesterol, which is known to be protective of heart health.

On the subject of heart health, you might be interested to know this: a high protein diet also reduces blood levels of an amino acid called homocysteine. Homocysteine is an established risk factor for cardiovascular disease and heart failure; elevated levels are also implicated in dementia. It is now recognised that people at risk of cardiovascular disease also have an increased risk of developing Alzheimer's. What links these two diseases is elevated homocysteine. What lowers homocysteine are certain B vitamins, namely folate, B12 and B6. Giving patients these vitamins in supplement form has been found to significantly reduce homocysteine levels. You do not need to supplement B vitamins if you eat enough meat. However non-meat eaters may need to supplement B12 as this vitamin is only found in animal-based foods – a fact that speaks volumes about human dietary requirements.

The trend towards high protein diets for weight loss has raised concerns over potential health effects, with particular regard to possible kidney damage. This concern is purely hypothetical: a review of the scientific literature on the subject found no evidence of any detrimental effects of a high protein intake on kidney function, except where there is an existing underlying metabolic abnormality. Nor has a high protein diet been found to induce bone loss, another hypothetical concern – quite the contrary, in fact. Deficiency of protein, even where there is sufficient calcium and vitamin D, can cause rapid change in bone density, as seen in osteoporosis. This is hardly surprising, as protein is a key nutrient for bone health and constitutes about a third of bone mass. Large studies suggest that high protein diets are associated with increased bone density and reduced incidence of osteoporotic fractures.

The fact that a high protein diet has not been found to have detrimental effects on health should come as no surprise. Protein is what ensured the survival of your lean and fit hunter-gatherer ancestors, despite the brutalities of the Ice Age. They ate a lot more protein (and fat) than we do today, and we know from the fossil record that they enjoyed far greater bone density. They certainly ate plenty of meat. The first modern humans emerged from Africa, and we know from analyses of bones and teeth that the diet they ate – the original *Homo sapiens* diet - was around 50 per cent plant based and 50 per cent animal based, with fish and shellfish comprising a significant portion of the animal component. I would suggest that this is the true meaning of a balanced diet.

(11) Say no whey

There is one source of animal protein that you should keep to a minimum, and that is milk. Even though milk has a low glycaemic index, and contains only a little carbohydrate (in the form of lactose), it is highly insulinotropic, meaning it stimulates the secretion of insulin, which in turn promotes the accumulation of body fat. The reason for this is the whey component. Whey is a protein that causes substantial spikes in insulin, although why and how it does this remains unknown. Therefore following *The Body Clock Diet* means excluding milk, yogurt and cream. A small splash of milk a couple of times a day in your tea is unlikely to have any effect, but hold the lattes and the cappuccinos. Cheese lovers will be thrilled and relieved to learn that most cheeses contain no whey and therefore have a rightful place on this programme, assuming you do not have an allergy or sensitivity to this food. Because whey is drawn off during the cheese making process, the finished product has a low insulin index. There is an exception, which is ricotta cheese, a product made from whey. Cottage cheese also contains some whey, but why would anyone want to eat this poor excuse for a cheese? Butter is also – thankfully - acceptable because it contains no whey, and is virtually pure fat.

(12) Get your timing right (part 2)

Once lunch is over, allow at least five hours before having your evening meal. The quality protein component of your lunch will ensure you feel satisfied all afternoon and can enjoy a good long stretch before you need to refuel.

Like lunch, dinner should consist of a protein component, with two portions of vegetables. These vegetables should be light with a very low carbohydrate content. You will soon be going to bed, and as your body is getting ready for some serious nocturnal fat combustion, it is especially important to keep your carbohydrate intake low.

Low to very low carbohydrate vegetables

Asparagus
Aubergine
Runner beans
Broccoli
Cabbage ·
Cauliflower
Kale
Fennel
Leeks
Marrow
Mushrooms
Green peppers
Pumpkin
Spinach
Spring greens
Watercress
Lettuce
Celery
Chicory
Cucumber
Tomato

I recommend that at least one of your two portions should be steamed greens. Steamed greens – spinach, broccoli, Swiss chard, that sort of thing - are ideal. They have a high water content but also a high fibre and magnesium content. Magnesium is the mineral that aids relaxation and sleep, and sleep promotes weight loss. Embellish with some black pepper and a generous knob of butter.

(13) Eat your greens (and reds, blues, yellows...)

We've established that you have to minimise insulin secretion, and avoid insulin resistance, in order to avoid gaining weight. Both these goals require that you avoid unnecessary carbohydrates. There are, however, some exceptions to the carb case. Fruit and vegetables pass muster not only because they have a low carbohydrate content and are 'good for you', they also, quite significantly, promote weight loss. This outcome is due to the presence of natural chemicals, or phytochemicals, found in plant foods. So there are no excuses at all for skipping your morning fruit or your lunch and evening vegetables.

There are two main groups of phytochemicals: carotenoids and polyphenols. Carotenoids are found in red, yellow and orange plant foods and this group includes carrots, tomatoes, peaches and apricots. They are also found in leafy green vegetables such as spinach and kale (the orange pigment is camouflaged by the dominant green). Polyphenols are found in darker plant foods, such as plums and berries, but are also found in red onions, green tea and mushrooms. Research suggests that these phytochemicals work as effective anti-obesity agents by suppressing the growth of adipose tissue and reducing fat mass. Phytochemicals are thought to alter fat cell metabolism and reduce the inflammation that can lead to insulin resistance and the metabolic syndrome. The adipose tissue which stores your fat is also the largest endocrine organ in the body and secretes a number of pro-inflammatory chemicals known as cytokines and adipokines. The more fat you have, the more inflammation you produce. This inflammation contributes to the development of insulin resistance and type 2 diabetes. The phytochemicals in fruits and vegetables have anti-inflammatory properties which target fat, reducing inflammation and fat mass, so form an essential part of your weight loss toolkit.

Eat fat to burn fat

When you eat a low carbohydrate diet you have to replace your usual carbs with something else. That something else is protein and fat. We've discussed protein; now you need to understand the importance of fat. There is no need to fear fat; it is your friend.

Your goal is to burn the surplus fat that resides in your adipose tissue. This fat, deposited around your belly, backside, hips and (insert here) may appear inert, but is in fact highly active. Fat moves in and out of your fuel depots all the time in the form of fatty acids, and it is this form that is used as fuel.

There are various kinds of body fat, but broadly speaking

there are two main types that form your energy reservoir: visceral and subcutaneous. Visceral fat occupies the abdominal area, and subcutaneous fat lies under your skin everywhere else. Most body fat – 80 per cent, approximately – is subcutaneous. Subcutaneous fat absorbs fatty acids more readily than visceral fat, hence its inelegant moniker 'metabolic sink.' Visceral fat has more hormone receptors and absorbs more glucose than subcutaneous fat. It also synthesizes inflammatory proteins more readily than visceral fat. It is this inflammation which can lead to the metabolic syndrome.

The combination of all these factors makes visceral fat a greater health hazard than subcutaneous fat. Men generally have more visceral fat (10-20 per cent of total fat) than women (5-8 per cent). However, visceral fat increases with age in both men and women, so it's never too soon to minimise its territory.

There's no fooling your body

Surplus energy is stored for a reason: to be drawn on when necessary. The trick is to make it necessary, and encourage your body's hormones and enzymes to facilitate the smooth passage of fatty acids out of your adipose tissue and into your blood, and from blood to all the cells in your body to burn for energy. Because you cannot fool your body's ancient bio-mechanisms that have evolved to conserve fuel whenever food intake is restricted, your cunning plan is to work with your biological programming, not against it. The whole point of this book is to show you how to burn that fat as efficiently as possible, without suffering health consequences or making your life a misery.

All that guff you may have heard about carbohydrate being the body's 'preferred' fuel is utter nonsense. Your body will always burn carbohydrate first, not because it loves it more but because circulating glucose is potentially lethal if it is not dealt with immediately. And this is how carbohydrates make you fat and keep you fat: for as long as you have available carbohydrate, in the form of glucose, circulating in your blood vessels, you will not burn the fat stored in your reservoirs – there's no need. As long as you continue to eat carbohydrates, your body will never have to dip into its fat reserves. When you eat fat it too will be stored as fat, *unless there is no glucose available* - in which case your body is only too happy to burn it. So, let's eat fat in order to burn fat.

Ketones for brains

When your diet is predominantly protein and fat you switch from burning glucose to burning fatty acids and chemicals called ketones. Fatty acids, as you saw above, are taken from your adipose tissue. They are perfectly adequate for most of the body to use for fuel, with the brain being an important exception. In the absence of glucose the brain will burn ketone bodies.

Ketone bodies are made in the liver, either from the fat we have eaten or from the fat we have stored. If required, they can also be made from certain amino acids. After a period of fasting, for example in the morning when you wake up, you are in a state of ketosis – you have raised levels of ketones in your blood. (Ketosis should not be confused (but often is, even by experts) with ketoacidosis, a pathological condition that can occur in diabetes when there is a shortage of insulin.) A low carbohydrate, high fat diet is sometimes referred to as a ketogenic diet. A ketogenic diet reduces insulin secretion and promotes weight loss.

Ketones provide energy for the brain and nervous system and fatty acids provide fuel for the rest of the body. Do not underestimate the importance of making ketones for your brain. The human brain is extremely demanding. Despite occupying only two per cent of body mass, it burns a whopping 20-25 per cent of the energy you consume – it needs around 400 calories a day to carry out its metabolic activities. That's before you even move a muscle. So just loafing about thinking about what you should be doing is a proactive, fat burning exercise in itself.

Once you are making ketones and burning fatty acids for energy your requirement for glucose is much reduced. Even during exercise ketosis can meet the metabolic demands of the body without it having to break down lean muscle. Studies consistently demonstrate that a low carbohydrate, ketogenic diet, consumed for more than seven days, markedly increases the rate of fat burning in exercisers, and enhances exercise performance, especially ultra-endurance exercise.

There is no official consensus on the correct level of carbohydrate restriction required to induce ketosis, although a daily diet of no more than 50 grams of carbs is considered effective. Which is fortunate, because by following *The Body Clock Diet* you will be consuming fewer than 50 grams of carbohydrate a day.

Eat the right kind of fat

We need to get more specific at this point because in fat world, there is fat, and then there is fat.

So, now that you can see that you are far better off, all round, on a high protein and fat, low carbohydrate diet (hurrah!), you need to know precisely what sort of fat to eat. This is a key issue. Some fats promote weight loss better than others, and some fats are so heinous that they negate the health benefits of a low carbohydrate diet, and even promote weight gain. The calories in fat were definitely not all created equal.

Despite the exponential growth of the obesity crisis over the last few decades, there has been no significant increase in the amount of fat people consume. Indeed, we eat less saturated fat than in the past, because for years now we've been told to consume 'healthy' polyunsaturated fats instead – margarines and spreads instead of butter, for example. Many people have, dutifully, complied. We've also been exhorted, quite emphatically, to consume low fat products such as skimmed milk and flavourless yogurts. We eat less fat, yet carry more body fat than ever before. We are also experiencing more chronic illness - heart disease, cancer and diabetes – despite eating all those 'heart-healthy' polyunsaturated fats. There's no mystery behind this figment of fattiness: as usual, you have been misinformed and misguided.

Oh my omega

This is what you need to know about polyunsaturated fats.

Briefly, there are two main families of polyunsaturates – omega-6 and omega-3. These two families are metabolically and functionally distinct; one cannot substitute the other.

The omega-6 fats are widely found in seeds and their oils, most commonly sunflower, safflower and sesame. Corn and soya oils are also high in omega-6 fatty acids. Perhaps you use these vegetable oils in your cooking. Perhaps you even use those much-hyped spreads instead of butter. Unfortunately, it is these omega-6, polyunsaturated fatty acids, masquerading as healthy options, which can make you fat.

The obesity epidemic has coincided with a marked increase in the consumption of omega-6 fatty acids, leading scientists to believe that there may be a cause and effect relationship. Indeed, plenty of recent studies have demonstrated that feeding omega-6 oils to animals increases fat mass and contributes to the metabolic syndrome. A high omega-6 diet triggers over-production of insulin, which in turn promotes fat storage. Feeding rats with soya oil, which is especially high in omega-6, has been shown to induce insulin resistance and insulin secretion failure. In one study, rats that were fed soya bean oil gained more body fat, and became more insulin resistant, than rats fed any other oil. As it happens, because the soya bean is an intensively farmed cash crop, soya bean oil is one of the most commonly consumed oils (by humans) worldwide.

There's more than weight gain to worry about with these oils. Once ingested, omega-6 oils are metabolised to powerful, hormone-like substances including prostaglandins and leukotrienes. Some of these are highly pro-inflammatory and in excessive amounts are believed to promote many modern diseases, including heart disease, cancer and arthritis.

From bad to worse

It gets worse, I'm afraid. These oils undergo a refining process involving high temperature treatment, bleaching and degumming before being incorporated into ready-meals, takeaways, margarines – everything and anything that is processed. These treatments denude the oil of any goodness they may once have contained, leaving notoriously harmful trans fatty acids in their place. That tub of hummus, or taramasalata, or jar of mayonnaise or sun-dried tomatoes - just about anything that contains oil - that you thought was so healthy, is instead chock-full of refined vegetable oils, loaded with omega-6 and trans fatty acids. Crisps, bread, biscuits … take a look at the ingredients lists. You'll find more omega-6 than you can shake a celery stick at. Critics of processed food are given to singling out saturated fat as one of the most heinous of ingredients, warning consumers that the junkiest of junk foods are full of it. They aren't, because saturated fat (butter, cream, milk) is relatively expensive. Instead they are full of cheap, nasty, refined omega-6 fats.

It is important to remember that both omega-6 and omega-3 oils are essential to health, but in the right amount and in their unrefined form. Consumption of omega-6 polyunsaturated fatty acids has soared in the major industrialised nations of the western world over the last few decades. This is evident even in human breast milk, which analyses show has seen a marked increase in omega-6 fatty acid content. Alongside this rapid increase in omega-6 fat intake there has been a parallel decrease in the consumption of omega-3 fatty acids, leading to a massive shift in ratio between the two groups. There is substantial evidence to suggest that we evolved on a diet containing equal amounts of omega-3 and omega-6 fatty acids. However, our highly processed, modern diets have tipped the ratio and we now get a staggering 15-16 times more omega-6 than omega-3. That's not good, and is a fast track to weight gain and ill health.

A different kettle of fish

Omega-3 fatty acids are in a different league altogether. Not only will these fats make you super healthy, they will also encourage your body to burn more of your stored fat. Yet these are the very oils most people consume so little of.

I am of course talking about oily fish, the most superior source of omega-3 fatty acids. More specifically, fish is the only meaningful dietary source of two fatty acids that belong to this family: EPA (eicosapentaenoic acid) and DHA (docosahexaenoic acid). These two fatty acids are essential for life, and as far as you are concerned, play a very important role in metabolism and weight loss. Mackerel, herring, sardines, salmon, trout, whitebait and anchovies are all rich in EPA and DHA.

Both animal and human studies suggest that omega-3 fatty acids can be very effective in helping to reduce overweight. They do this in a number of ways: they encourage fat oxidation, they suppress appetite and they shift metabolism away from fat accumulation and towards the building of lean tissue, thereby also improving body composition. Fish oil also promotes weight loss through its effect on insulin: it helps prevent insulin resistance and other metabolic disorders. A study published in 2010 in the *Journal of the International Society of Sports Nutrition* reported that when a group of men and women were given either fish oil or safflower oil supplements (a significant source of omega-6) for a period of six weeks, without the participants knowing which supplement they were taking, or changing their diets in any way, only those taking the fish oil experienced a significant reduction in fat mass and an increase in lean muscle.

EPA and DHA are also crucial for brain function, and let's not forget that the human brain burns around 400 calories a day to meet its metabolic needs. The very large human brain, which is made predominantly of fat, depends on polyunsaturated fatty acids, and in particular DHA; there is more DHA in the brain than any other fatty acid.

In short, you need to reduce your intake of omega-6 fats and increase your intake of omega-3 fats. Omega-6 fats are essential to life, in moderation and in their natural unrefined form, and you can easily meet your requirements by consuming meat, nuts and seeds. But like most people, you probably need to seriously increase your intake of oily fish. I advise two to three portions weekly.

Super saturated

As well as eating plenty of oily fish, you will also need to include saturated fat in your weight loss regime. There is, after all, only so much oily fish you can eat and you are not a seal. As you saw earlier, fat does not make you fat, and a low carbohydrate, high fat diet is much more effective than a low fat, high carbohydrate diet. Saturated fat is a great medium for cooking (butter and coconut oil are saturated fats). It also makes foods palatable and filling. Quite frankly, saturated fat makes food utterly delicious, and, as luck would have it, forms part of the healthy diet on which we evolved to our present form.

Saturated fat has been part of the human diet since the *Homo* genus swung down from the trees and landed on the wide-open savannahs of Africa and saw that it was full of large game. It served us perfectly well, for around 2.5 million years, and was never considered detrimental to human health until the 1960s when *Homo expertus* emerged, clutching a clipboard and telling us that for the entire history of humanity we'd been doing it all wrong. Since then, and despite any real evidence to substantiate the litany of dire warnings, saturated fat has been branded a killer. It makes you wonder how on earth we survived for over two million years.

We obviously did survive, despite our high fat, low margarine diet. Nutrition scientists have long been baffled by the absence of heart disease, cancer and other 'diseases of civilisation' observed in modern hunter-gatherer societies such as the Hadza who live in the Lake Eyasi region of Northern Tanzania, and who even today persist with their high fat, high meat diets.

Miscarriage of justice

Again, what appears to be a paradox is just something that debunks a preconceived idea. Saturated fat does not cause heart disease, but excessive carbohydrates and refined omega-6 fats do, as the research consistently demonstrates. When a low fat diet was compared to a low carbohydrate diet over a period of twelve weeks, after being consumed by forty subjects considered at risk of cardiovascular disease, not only did the low carbohydrate group show more favourable results – lower glucose and insulin - they also experienced ten per cent more weight loss, *despite a threefold higher intake of saturated fat*. A raft of similar studies has demonstrated similar results; consequently in 2010 researchers writing in the journal *Nutrition* state that there is little evidence to support long-standing dietary recommendations to eat a low fat, high carbohydrate diet, and ask whether these recommendations should continue or *whether there might not be better alternatives*.

The fact is that vast amounts of evidence have accrued showing that saturated fat has little or no causal effect on heart disease, yet this evidence continues to be ignored. Even the World Health Organization, after studying all the research, concluded that '*there is no probable or convincing evidence for significant effects of total dietary fats on coronary heart disease or cancers... There is **probable** evidence that replacing SFA (saturated fatty acids) with largely refined carbohydrates has no benefit on CHD, (coronary heart disease) and may even increase the risk of CHD.*' Those same experts found that although there was a strong link between fish oil and reduced risk of heart disease, dietary saturated fat was not significantly associated with heart disease or mortality. Their conclusion was that *There is probably no direct relation between total fat intake and risk of CHD.*

So, you can stop worrying and instead focus on weight loss, your main concern at this moment. There clearly are better alternatives, as those researchers suggested, which not only promote weight loss but do so without the hunger pangs and cravings associated with reduced calorie diets.

Grass-fed is best

It is my guess that you are more likely to cook your evening meal than any other meal, which is why it is so important not only to cook with the right kind of fat but to choose the right kind of protein. The right kind of protein – meat and fish - comes with a ready supply of fat. This is a perfect arrangement as fat not only makes food more palatable, it also prevents excessive protein consumption. Therefore feel free to enjoy lots of red meat, namely beef, lamb, pork and venison, but be aware that there is a world of difference between meat from intensively reared animals (which unfortunately is most meat on sale in supermarkets) and meat from free-range, grass-fed animals. Aside from the ethical and welfare issues (and they are legion), the main issue, in terms of health and weight, lies in the fat content.

Intensively reared animals are fed a diet that is not natural to them, high in grain and soya. Consequently, the meat is disproportionately high in omega-6 fats, the very fats that can facilitate weight gain. Grass-fed animals, on the other hand, tend to produce meat much higher in omega-3 and monounsaturated fatty acids (see below for more details on the benefits of monounsaturates).

Therefore, wherever and whenever you can, make sure you buy meat ethically produced from free-range, grass-fed livestock. The same applies to poultry and eggs. It's not only we humans who are what we eat.

King coconut

An oil that not only cooks your food beautifully but also actively speeds up weight loss sounds like a fanciful notion, but may I present coconut oil, the multi-tasker of the larder. Terribly trendy at the moment, coconut is deserving of its elevated culinary status. It is rich in medium-chain fatty acids, and it is these fatty acids (also found to a lesser extent in butter and palm oil) that have been the focus of a considerable amount of research in the weight loss area. In particular, both human and animal studies have demonstrated enhanced thermogenesis (increased metabolic rate) and accelerated fat oxidation after consumption of medium-chain fatty acids. Trials have also found that these fatty acids have a greater satiating effect than other oils. Furthermore, they improve insulin sensitivity and reduce the risk of developing metabolic syndrome.

When it comes to testing coconut at the coalface, there are plenty of studies to choose from, but here's one that's fairly typical. When forty women were divided into two groups and given either 30mls of soya bean oil or 30mls of coconut oil over a twelve week period, but otherwise followed the same diet and did the same amount of exercise, only the group given coconut oil demonstrated significant weight loss and health benefits by the end of the trial. Notably, they experienced a reduction in waist circumference, and blood tests revealed raised HDL and lowered LDL cholesterol – a status considered protective of heart health. The soya bean group (soya being exceptionally high in omega-6 fat) had no such luck with their waist circumferences or HDL status.

Like olive oil (see below), when buying coconut oil you should seek out cold-pressed virgin coconut oil (VCO) which is made from fresh coconut kernel, dried in the sun or on a low heat. Avoid copra, which is industrially produced, refined coconut oil whose nutritional value is negligible compared to VCO.

The virtuous extra virgin

Alongside saturated fat, there is also a place for monounsaturated fat in your weight loss programme. The best known source of monounsaturated fat is olive oil, although red meat also contains significant quantities. Olive oil is perfectly acceptable on this programme, as it does not produce the harmful effects created by excessive omega-6 oils. What's more, monounsaturated fat can help control blood sugar levels and prevent abdominal fat accumulation.

When it comes to cooking, and salad dressing, you can be quite liberal with olive oil, but it must be of the extra virgin variety. If it isn't extra virgin it's just plain olive oil, which means it has undergone intense processing, including high heat treatment, degumming, bleaching and deodorisation, processes which remove any trace of original nutritional goodness. Extra virgin olive is cold-pressed, and by law cannot be subjected to the intense refinement of ordinary olive oil.

Sup up your soup

Here's a top tip for dinner: soup. Soup satisfies without leaving you feeling stuffed. Studies have regularly shown that soup is more filling than solid food. The explanation for this has always eluded researchers, but when subjects were actually tested for gastric emptying (that's the term, honest, to describe the speed at which food leaves your stomach) after consuming either a solid meal, a chunky soup or a smooth soup, they discovered something rather interesting. The longest gastric emptying time occurred after consuming smooth soup and the shortest after the solid meal – meaning that the volunteers felt fullest after the smooth soup. It may be time to buy yourself one of those nifty hand-held blenders, if you haven't already got one.

This meal is your flexible friend; you can throw into the pot any assortment of leftovers or stray vegetables you find lurking in the fridge and whizz them up. Make sure you add meat or fish (not blended, obviously) for your protein component. This is a gloriously hearty meal, so make the most of it during the cold season. Personally, I think there's nothing quite like a hot chicken and vegetable soup on a cold winter's night.

 Drink the right alcohol, in the right amount

Because one gram of alcohol contains seven calories, it has usually been assumed, quite reasonably, that alcohol consumption may contribute to weight gain. However, this is a surprisingly unclear area. Alcohol is not stored in the body, and because it is potentially toxic the body prioritises its oxidation. A review of the best quality studies of the subject – thirty-one – found that there was no clear, conclusive evidence of a positive association between alcohol consumption and weight gain when consumed in light to moderate quantities. Furthermore, research has shown that insulin resistance is less likely to occur in individuals with regular light to moderate alcohol consumption (always light to moderate!) but more likely to occur in heavy drinkers (four or more drinks a day). Moderate alcohol consumption improves insulin sensitivity and is associated with a lower risk of developing diabetes and the metabolic syndrome. Anything that improves insulin sensitivity also reduces the risk of weight gain. Daily consumption of fewer than 40 grams of alcohol by men, and 20 grams by women, significantly reduces the prevalence of metabolic syndrome. Again, this quantity represents moderate intake. In the UK, one unit of alcohol (10ml) is equal to 8 grams. A 175ml glass of red wine contains 2 units. To be on the safe side, I recommend that men limit their alcohol intake to maximum three units of alcohol a day and women to two.

Red before bed

When you do partake, make yours a glass of red wine. Red wine is special because it contains a natural chemical called resveratrol, which has been found to have the glorious effect of inhibiting something called *de novo lipogenesis* – the creation of fat from dietary carbohydrate. It not only decreases the creation of fat, it can also alter fat mass and improve insulin sensitivity in fat cells. In numerous studies of diabetic rats, resveratrol has been found to reduce blood insulin and blood sugar. The few studies that have been carried out on humans have produced similar results, which is very encouraging.

Takeaway

- Snacking between meals is unnecessary and will inhibit fat burning
- Protein suppresses appetite and increases satiety
- Protein increases resting metabolic rate and encourages fat oxidation
- A high protein diet is a healthy diet, and is the one to which the human body is genetically adapted
- Milk, cream and yogurt should be avoided as they contain whey, a protein that causes spikes in insulin
- Eating fat does not make you fat
- As long as you continue to eat lots of carbohydrates, you will not burn body fat
- When carbohydrates are not available, your body switches to burning fatty acids and ketones from your body fat
- Refined omega-6 polyunsaturated oils promote weight gain
- Omega-3 fatty acids, as found in oily fish, promote weight loss
- Saturated fat forms part of the natural human diet
- Coconut oil, a saturated fat, can aid weight loss

Takeaway continued
- Extra virgin olive oil can help maintain even blood sugar and prevent fat accumulation
- Meat from grass-fed animals is higher in omega-3 fats and monounsaturates, and meat from intensively farmed animals is higher in omega-6 fats
- Low to moderate amounts of alcohol, especially red wine, can help prevent weight gain

Part Five

BEDTIME. YOU THOUGHT IT WAS ALL OVER? IT'S ONLY JUST BEGUN

Understanding the interaction between circadian and metabolic systems might ultimately contribute to the design of improved rational therapies, not only for sleep disturbances, but also for obesity and diabetes mellitus. (Kohsaka and Bass 2006)

(18) Sleep it off

It makes sense to eat a good protein meal with light vegetables in the evening because your body switches to burning fatty acids and ketones during sleep. However, if your stomach is full of food waiting to be digested, that happy arrangement will be delayed. During the day, we metabolise food faster, and it passes through the gut faster; eating late at night is more likely to lead to weight gain. For that same reason, ensure that you have finished eating at least three hours before retiring to bed.

If you eat at around 6pm in the evening, and don't eat breakfast until 9am the following morning, you will have fasted for 15 hours. Fasting – or intermittent fasting, as it is known - confers many health benefits, including improved brain and heart function. It is also an effective weight loss strategy and its success has been documented in research since the 1940s. There are several types of fasting methods, but an extended overnight fast is by far the easiest and is highly effective when combined with eating the right foods right time, which of course is what you are doing on *The Body Clock Diet*.

Tick tock

Now it's time to take into consideration another pivotal element of your internal body clock. When and how long you sleep, and the frequency and timing of your meals, can all influence the way your body burns or stores your food, so you need to ensure you are aligned with, and not against, this powerful timekeeper. The circadian rhythm (circadian in Latin means 'about a day') is an ancient inner clock, which functions with near twenty-four hour precision. Located in the hypothalamic suprachiasmatic nucleus region of the brain, this biological clock is mysterious, and more than a little otherworldly. It responds to the rising and setting of the sun so that our patterns of sleep and wakefulness match the rotation of the Earth about its axis. It was Charles Darwin who, after visiting the Galapagos Islands in 1835, first realised that life is cyclical, and he later published a treatise on the daily pattern of leaf movements in plants. It is well known now that this invisible clock ticks in most animals too.

Any disruption to this biological timekeeper can have serious consequences for metabolism and hormone secretion. Much of this disruption has been blamed on electric lighting and the 24-hour lifestyle to which we have grown accustomed. We create our own, dissonant settings, which ultimately clash with our clocks and create disharmony in our hormones. The phenomenon of living against the clock has been termed 'social jetlag' by scientists, and this form of jetlag has been found to significantly increase the likelihood of being overweight; conversely, adequate sleep has been found to reduce that likelihood. Work and school timetables, and the use of alarm clocks to align wakefulness with those timetables, contribute to the amount of social jetlag accrued by each individual. Social jetlag is at its most extreme during adolescence (they really do need to stay in bed half the morning) but continues throughout the working life.

The whole world is getting fatter - prevalence of obesity across the globe has doubled since 1980 – and at the same time, there has been a parallel trend in reduced sleep duration. There is growing and convincing evidence that the two phenomena are linked. Consider the US, where obesity is an even bigger crisis than it is here in the UK (but we're catching up fast). Americans are sleeping less. A 1960 survey conducted by the American Cancer Society found that on average people most commonly enjoyed between eight and nine hours sleep a night. Fast-forward to 1995, when another survey, this time by the National Sleep Foundation, found that sleeping for seven hours was the norm. More recently, research has found that six or fewer hours is common.

The majority of studies (and there have been around 50 worldwide) looking at the link between sleep and obesity in adults and children have found a significant association between short sleep duration (less than six hours) and increased risk of obesity. Duration of six or fewer hours has also been associated with other health problems, such as diabetes. Every night, as you sleep, your body balances its energy accounts and in the morning you wake up and discover how the books are looking. So now you've finished eating - and spent the evening relaxing for at least three hours - it's time to go to bed to luxuriate in those seven to eight hours of blissful, fat-burning sleep.

While you were sleeping...

Your metabolic rate falls by around 15 per cent during sleep. If you think about it, this is a surprisingly small reduction for such apparent inertia. But don't be deceived; as you slumber, blissfully unaware of the workings of your autonomic nervous system, your body is busy carrying out innumerable metabolic processes, and your brain is burning fuel furiously. The human brain consumes in the region of 20 per cent of what you eat, and approximately *16 times more than muscle*. No wonder thinking hard can be so exhausting. It's like an intense cerebral workout. Your brain is a fuel-hungry furnace, demanding around 400 calories a day.

Look after your brain, and it will repay you in kind. Sleep for seven to eight hours, in a darkened room, and your brain will switch on the hormones that initiate fat burning. At night, when you are in fasting mode, growth hormone (GH) swings into action. This noble, fat-mobilising hormone stimulates the production of ketones and the release of fatty acids from your fat stores to provide your brain and the rest of your body with the fuel needed to perform innumerable metabolic functions. The secretion of GH starts at the beginning of the first deep sleep cycle. However, peak GH secretion is inhibited if the onset of sleep is delayed.

GH is, in a way, the opposite of insulin. Whereas insulin

is the dominant hormone during and after meals, GH is dominant during fasting at night. Lack of GH at this time increases muscle protein breakdown and can result in increased fat mass; all the more reason to take yourself off to bed in good time. The sooner you go to bed, the sooner your GH can get to work.

Leptin love

Sleep influences the regulation of two other hormones involved in fat metabolism: leptin and ghrelin. You read about ghrelin in part three - it is secreted in the stomach and stimulates appetite by acting as a hunger signal to the brain. Levels of ghrelin rise during calorie restriction, hence the gnawing hunger of a low calorie diet. Leptin (from the Greek word *leptos* meaning thin) acts in opposition to ghrelin. It is essentially an appetite suppressant; it is secreted by fat cells and informs the brain that they do not require more fat.

Leptin communicates with the brain, passing on information about energy requirements. It peaks when you are asleep, which explains why you might go to bed on an empty stomach but do not (unless you have a metabolic disturbance) wake up hungry in the middle of the night.

It is in your interest to allow leptin to get on with its job; however, if you don't get enough sleep, it can't. Instead, there will be a reversal of roles: sleep deprivation causes ghrelin to rise, and leptin to fall. There is an interesting piece of research that has been ongoing since 1993, called the Wisconsin Sleep Cohort Study. One notable finding to emerge from this continuous research is that a loss of three hours sleep (five hours instead of eight) is associated with low leptin, high ghrelin and an average four to five per cent greater body weight.

The rule, therefore, is to not let anything stand in the way of you and your leptin production. Make sure you get enough sleep, and avoid calorie restriction. If you restrict calorie intake, leptin levels fall rapidly. This sends a message to the brain to eat more and restrict energy expenditure. That is why a low calorie diet can make you feel tired and disinclined to engage in physical activity.

(19) Don't be a night owl

Unfortunately, it's not just lack of sleep that can lead to weight gain; so too can sleeping at the wrong time. When mice, which are nocturnal mammals, are fed during the day (when they would normally be asleep) they gain significantly more weight than mice fed only during the night, when they are normally awake and feeding. The same has been found in rats, which are prone to obesity when given food at a time when they would normally be asleep. Human shift workers are no different: studies consistently show that overweight and obesity are far more prevalent in shift workers than day workers, and that shift work is a risk factor for becoming overweight. I'm sorry to say that there is no solution to this issue if you are a shift worker; I can only advise that you make sure that you still get seven to eight hours of unbroken sleep, and in a darkened room.

The order of the day

1. Substantial breakfast when hungry
2. Fruit - just before breakfast and/or lunch (two pieces in total)
3. Lunch – four hours after finishing breakfast
4. Dinner – five hours after finishing lunch. Small handful of nuts or olives half an hour or less before dinner, if required
5. Bed, three hours or more after dinner
6. 7-8 hours sleep in a darkened room

Takeaway

- The evening meal should be eaten three hours or more before bed
- An extended overnight fast can make a valuable contribution to weight loss
- The brain houses an ancient metabolic clock, which when disrupted upsets the hormones which govern metabolism
- Living against the clock can cause obesity
- During deep sleep growth hormone ensures you switch to burning fatty acids and ketones from your fat stores
- Sleep deprivation results in weight gain
- Humans are meant to sleep at night and disruptions to this routine can result in weight gain

Part Six

ANY TIME, ANY PLACE: 24/7

(20) Check your thermostat

I saw a woman wearing a sweatshirt with Guess on it.
I said, Thyroid problem? Arnold Schwarzenegger

There are some aspects of metabolism which apply to any time of the day or night. Thyroid function is one of them. No matter how good your diet, or how much you exercise, it'll all come to nothing if your thyroid is functioning below par. This is the master gland that governs every aspect of metabolism, and it demands respect.

The thyroid is a gland at the front of the neck, shaped rather like a butterfly and consisting of two lobes, one on either side of the windpipe. It oversees metabolism in virtually every cell of the body and is responsible for your basal metabolic rate, the rate at which you burn food when at rest. Metabolic activity creates heat, so the thyroid is also responsible for maintaining body temperature. So if you don't produce enough thyroid hormone, you may find you put on weight all too easily, and feel cold even when it isn't.

It all starts in the brain, which produces thyroid-stimulating hormone (TSH), which in turn stimulates the production of thyroxine (*aka* T4 because it contains four atoms of iodine) and triiodothyronine (*aka* T3 because it contains three atoms of iodine). T4 is converted to T3, its active form. Thyroid hormone is the term used to describe both these hormones together.

Under the weather

If you have an underactive thyroid, you have a condition known as hypothyroidism. The most noticeable symptom is weight gain that is stubbornly hard to shift. But as this is the master gland, controlling all aspects of metabolism, chances are you will also experience low energy, mental apathy, feeling cold all the time and even constipation. It's as if everything grinds to a halt; it's all too much and you really can't be bothered.

What causes hypothyroidism? One of the best ways to abuse your thyroid is through yo-yo dieting – yet another reason to avoid punitive, calorie-restricted weight loss programmes. A significant reduction in food intake slows down your metabolic rate – or more specifically, slows down the activity of the thyroid gland. Because your Stone-Age body is programmed to do its damnedest to retain fat reserves when food intake is restricted, it does. As calorie intake falls, so too does the level of thyroid hormone output. Calorie restriction causes a reduction in T3 production, and eventually you find that you have to eat less and less just to stay at the same weight. You can only keep this up for so long, as every hard-boiled dieter will concur. This system evolved over millennia as a defence mechanism against famine and you are very much deluded if you think you can beat it. 'Underfeeding', as the scientific literature calls it, results in a reduction in metabolic rate. In one study of 144 morbidly obese patients, nearly twenty per cent were found to have either overt or subclinical hypothyroidism. So you might be suspicious if you have any of the symptoms given above, and even more so if you are overweight but not overeating, and have a history of yo-yo dieting. Remember those wretched Minnesota starvation volunteers?

Everything is connected

Another possible cause of hypothyroidism is metabolic syndrome, as described in part three. The two conditions are very much related, which is not as bad as it sounds because when you correct metabolic syndrome you can expect improvement in thyroid function. When 278 subjects with metabolic syndrome were compared with 261 subjects free of the condition, it was found that those with metabolic syndrome had higher TSH levels. When someone has high levels of TSH it usually means that their thyroid is underactive, as extra TSH is being pumped out in an attempt to stimulate more thyroid hormone. Other studies have similarly found that people with metabolic syndrome have elevated TSH levels, and high TSH levels are associated with greater body mass index.

The best way to reduce your chance of developing metabolic syndrome is by controlling blood sugar levels, and by doing so you also increase levels of thyroid hormone. Imagine how positively this affects your health, as well as your waistline. When a group of twelve men switched from a diet containing 48 per cent carbohydrate to a diet containing just eight per cent carbohydrate, they not only experienced a whopping 34 per cent drop in blood insulin and a significant decrease in fat mass – 3.4 kilos – they also experienced an 11 percent increase in total thyroxine.

Iodine: thyroid fuel

Several nutrients play an important role in the smooth

running of the thyroid, but none so much as iodine, which makes up over half the weight of thyroid hormone. Iodine is found in seafood, seaweed (where it was first discovered), dairy foods (not naturally; it is routinely added to cattle feed), some vegetables and anything that contains iodized salt. Iodine deficiency is a major cause of hypothyroidism worldwide. When deficiency is severe, so are the consequences, especially for growth and development. During pregnancy and early infancy, iodine deficiency can result in cretinism, an irreversible condition characterized by stunted growth and mental disability. Iodine deficiency is recognised by the World Health Organization as the most common preventable cause of brain damage in the world today.

That pesky Ice Age

The scale of the problem is due to the fact that most of the iodine on the planet is in the sea, not soil. One of the main causes of soil depletion is the glaciation that occurred during the last ice age, which exposed the iodine-rich layers of soil to rain, flooding and wind, all of which washed iodine into the sea. Soil erosion has resulted in depletion of this crucial element, especially in areas that were once covered by glaciers.

Until recently, iodine deficiency was associated mainly with Asia and sub-Saharan Africa, but we know now that it is much more widespread. Because we obtain most of our iodine from seafood and dairy produce, anyone who avoids these foods might be at greater risk of deficiency. Therefore vegans and vegetarians are especially vulnerable. So too is anyone who avoids fish, which from what I can tell is the majority of people in the UK.

Data suggest that iodine deficiency is more common than generally believed. Although prevalence is not as severe as in developing countries, mild to moderate iodine deficiency is not uncommon across Europe. The more severe the deficiency, the more severe the deficiency disorders. A review of studies of pregnant women across Europe concluded that most women are iodine deficient, at least during their pregnancy.

The UK is no exception, and there is concern that many pregnant women here have low iodine status, putting their unborn child at risk of reduced intelligence and impaired motor skills. In 2013 the iodine status of 664 schoolgirls aged 14-15 across the UK was assessed by measuring urine levels. The results showed mild iodine deficiency in 51 per cent of the girls, moderate deficiency in 16 per cent and severe deficiency in 1 per cent. If the overwhelming majority of teenage girls are iodine deficient, there is every reason to assume that so too is the majority of everyone else in the UK. You may find it useful to test your iodine status. This test is not usually available on the NHS, but test kits are now available for purchase direct from medical laboratories on-line.

Beyond iodine: selenium, iron and zinc

The thyroid requires more than just iodine. Among the other nutrients it needs are selenium, iron and zinc.

There is a high concentration of the trace element selenium in the thyroid, because it is required for the conversion of T4 to T3. Like iodine, selenium shortage is recognised as a potentially serious issue. As long ago as

1997 an article in the British Medical Journal claimed it was *'time to act'* on the worrying depletion of selenium levels in soil throughout the world, including Europe. This article reported that 22 years previously, selenium intake in Britain was 60mcg daily, compared to 34mcg daily in 1997. Selenium is found in Brazil nuts (one of the richest sources), fish, seafood and meat (especially offal). The latest dietary survey on nutrient intake in the UK found that 87 per cent of adults were consuming less than the recommended intake (75 mcg daily for men and 60mcg for women).

Deficiency of iron and zinc could also lead to impaired thyroid function. Zinc is required for all hormone production, including thyroid hormone. Like selenium, it is required for the conversion of T4 to T3. Good sources include meat, especially red meat, fish and seafood.

Iron deficiency blunts the potency of iodine; it impairs thyroid metabolism by reducing levels of T4 and T3, an effect that has been demonstrated in both human and animal studies. The best source of iron is red meat. Iron from plant sources has poor bioavailability by comparison, meaning that very little is absorbed. So if you are vegetarian, it might be worth having a blood test for iron deficiency anaemia; you may have to supplement.

Testing times

If you suspect that your thyroid is functioning below par, the first thing you need to do is see your GP and get tested. If test results reveal that you do indeed have hypothyroidism, the standard treatment is thyroxine, which is given as a synthetic hormone called levothyroxine.

There are various tests that your GP can arrange, but bear in mind that even when test results come back 'normal', you can still have what is called mild, or sub-clinical hypothyroidism. Be sure that the test you undergo includes measurement of TSH. As you just read, elevated TSH levels alone may mean you have mild hypothyroidism as your body is having to work extra hard to produce enough thyroid hormone. The problem is compounded by the fact that different laboratories have different measurements of what is normal – if your test results are only just within the 'normal' range, you may still have borderline, subclinical hypothyroidism.

Sub-clinical hypothyroidism is believed by many experts to represent mild thyroid failure and, according to researchers writing in the *Journal of Clinical Endocrinology and Metabolism, 'is a clinically important disorder that has adverse clinical consequences that should be treated in most, if not all, cases'*. Quite; if you have sub-clinical hypothyroidism you may well experience all the symptoms of overt hypothyroidism, including weight gain.

Seaweed in the kitchen

In addition to Brazil nuts, red meat, fish and seafood, make edible seaweed part of your regular thyroid-friendly diet. Everyone needs iodine, and everyone is at risk of deficiency and needs to ensure regular intake. Sea vegetables are currently enjoying a welcome culinary comeback. They are a gift, as far as their mineral content is concerned. They lend themselves beautifully to soups, stews and stir fries, and because they are rich in sodium, you don't need to add any salt to the end product. Most importantly, edible seaweed is a great source of natural iodine.

If you are vegetarian, vegan or avoid dairy and seafood, I would suggest exploring edible seaweeds, if you don't already. The Japanese make good use of seaweeds, which over here were once the preserve of the hard-core health food store. Happily you can now buy them in most large supermarkets. Nori, kombu, dulse, wakame, arame and red seaweed (also known as carragheen) are perhaps the most commonly available seaweeds in the UK. It is not recommended that you start taking iodine in the form of seaweed supplements because if you over-consume iodine you may put yourself at risk of developing *hyperthyroidism*, or over-active thyroid disorder.

Foods to avoid (but only if you have thyroid trouble)

Certain foods contain substances called goitrogens, which are believed to enlarge the thyroid and cause hypothyroidism by blocking the conversion of T4 hormone to T3. They can also inhibit the body's ability to use iodine. Foods that contain goitrogens include the brassica family: kale, sprouts, cauliflower and cabbage. Other goitrogenic foods include soya, radishes, watercress, mustard, turnips, cassava and peanuts. However, don't panic. These foods only have this effect where there is an existing underactive thyroid disorder and/or iodine deficiency, and only applies to raw foods - cooking these foods disables the goitrogens they contain, so they become harmless. After all, many of us eat these worthy vegetables quite frequently, without developing thyroid problems. So if you have an underactive thyroid, avoid raw greens, but if you haven't, don't. Soya, being a bean, is not part of this programme, which is just as well as cooking does not disable the goitrogens in soya beans.

(21) Cool your jets

Future research needs to better define levels of risk and appropriate treatments based not only on one's girth but also on the multiple causes of central fat, such as genetics, behavior, general obesity, and chronic stress. (Epel et al 2000)

Stress can make you fat. It's bad enough that food can make you fat, without an abstract notion putting the boot in. Yet not only does stress mess with your mind, it messes with your body, impeding fat loss and actually promoting fat accumulation. Clearly then, you have to either get rid of the stress in your life, or prime your body to negate its harmful effects. Ideally, you'll do both.

The stress response to a potentially dangerous situation is a sublime example of evolutionary engineering at its best. Your heart pumps faster and you breathe faster, delivering oxygen to your muscles; blood gets ready to clot in case you are wounded. Your amazing, built-in stress response system ensures you have the speed and alertness to either put up a good fight or run for the hills. Unrelenting stress, on the other hand, the sort that doggedly persists for much longer than what might be considered normal, is not so amazing. It impedes hormone function and promotes weight gain. It's all about the cortisol.

Cortisol cycle

Adrenaline is a hormone released by the adrenal glands as a reaction to immediate, short-term stress, sometimes called the alarm stage. The hormone cortisol is also secreted by the adrenals, but as a reaction to prolonged stress. It's a hormone that also gives you energy. Normally, cortisol is produced cyclically as part of the circadian rhythm. In the healthy individual, levels of this hormone start to rise between 3 a.m. and 6 a.m. and gradually decrease throughout the day, so that by night-time it is at its lowest. With unrelenting stress, this system goes awry and cortisol is produced in excess and at the wrong time.

Cortisol does a number of things in relation to metabolism, including mobilising glucose for energy, thus increasing blood-sugar levels. And this is where, in excess, it turns from friend to foe. Unless you require a surge in sugar to fight or flee, which I'm assuming you don't, this blood sugar will be converted to fat and added to your existing fat store. Most likely it will be despatched to your abdominal region as this area is much more sensitive to cortisol than subcutaneous fat.

Belly fat sucks

Abdominal fat is different from other body fat. It has greater blood flow, and up to four times more cortisol receptors. Your belly just sucks it up. For this reason it is also a risk factor for hypertension, coronary heart disease, stroke and diabetes.

Both animal and human studies have confirmed that stress-induced cortisol secretion increases abdominal fat.

When fifty-nine healthy, premenopausal women were subjected to regular laboratory stress sessions over four days, they were assessed for cortisol and psychological responses. Sure enough, those women who coped less well with stress secreted significantly more cortisol and had higher levels of abdominal fat than those who coped better. That's because as cortisol levels rise, so too does insulin, and elevated cortisol exacerbates insulin resistance. Everything is connected, and nothing illustrates this more alarmingly than the knock-on effects of prolonged stress.

Even a reduced calorie diet is stressful and has indeed been found to increase cortisol levels. When women on a diet of 1,200 calories a day had their stress perception monitored and their salivary cortisol measured, it was found that restricting calories led to an increase in both perceived stress levels and total cortisol output.

Cortisol doesn't stop there, either, as part of its ploy to fatten you. Cortisol levels are naturally low in the evening as you prepare for sleep, but stress changes the natural order of things and forces your adrenals to keep pumping out cortisol in the evening. This impacts on other hormones, including growth hormone. You saw earlier that growth hormone is the key to burning fat stores during deep sleep. At night, elevated cortisol suppresses the secretion of growth hormone - so even sleep offers no respite as stress rolls on, leaving a trail of hormone havoc.

Craving comfort

Another problem, as many of you may have already noticed, is that stress makes you crave all the wrong foods and eat more of them. Animals have been observed to under-eat when stressed, but when offered highly palatable food such as lard and sugar combined, they will go for it.

Humans are rather similar. Some people decrease their food intake under stress but most consume more, possibly because of the range of 'palatable' foods such as chocolate that are so readily available to provide emotional support. Indeed, the foods most favoured by the fat and stressed are those with a high fat and/or sugar content. The fat of course is not the issue – but combine fat with sugar, as in chocolate, and you have the ideal comfort food. Most chocolate has the wrong type of fat too – vegetable fat, which is full of the omega-6 fatty acids which make a hefty contribution to weight gain. A study into eating behaviour, published in the journal *Health Psychology* in 2008, found, not surprisingly, that stress was associated with increased consumption of processed snacks and reduced consumption of main meals and vegetables.

Of rats and men

These comfort foods reach the reward centres of the brain in a way that other foods cannot, and they override the homeostatic signals that would normally tell you when enough is enough. When under stress, both humans and rats will eat when not hungry, and are unable to stop when they are full. Giving cortisol infusions has been found to induce increased food intake in both rats and humans (who are starting to look very similar). In research, stressed rats will happily expose themselves to cold or shock in order to get their comfort foods – peanut butter, sweets, chocolate chips. Funny enough, these foods are also rather attractive to stressed humans as they enhance mood and stimulate the reward centres of the brain, an effect seen in human brain imaging. It is these reward centres that largely determine what we eat when stressed, when unable to differentiate hunger cues from emotional arousal. In obese people, sadness and emotional distress are triggers for eating foods that combine fat and sugar, even in the absence of hunger.

Taming cortisol

Now for the good news: you might be stressed, but you can still manipulate cortisol secretion through diet. Of course you will also need to look at stress management, but there is a lot you can achieve just through making dietary changes. Fortunately, the first dietary approach that helps normalise cortisol focuses on regulating blood sugar levels, which is precisely what you are doing by following *The Body Clock Diet*. The next most significant alteration to your diet is the increased consumption of the fatty acids EPA and DHA, as found in oily fish. Low levels of these fatty acids are associated with over-stimulation of the stress response, and supplementing with fish oil has been found to inhibit adrenal activation triggered by mental stress. I recommend taking fish oil supplements on this programme if you suffer from prolonged stress, as it may be exacerbating your weight gain. Take two 1000mg capsules daily, one in the morning and one in the evening. Obviously you won't do this if you are allergic to fish. Fish oil supplements are also contraindicated if you take blood-thinning medication such as warfarin. Note that you should take fish oil, not cod liver oil. Cod liver oil is great for vitamins A and D, but not so great for EPA and DHA.

Healthy adrenal function also requires vitamin C, the vitamin B complex and the mineral magnesium. You will get plenty of vitamin C from your fruit and vegetable consumption on this programme, and B complex from meat and other animal-based foods. Magnesium deserves particular attention, because it is an important mineral for cortisol regulation, muscle relaxation and sleep. However, dietary intake in the western diet is considered inadequate. Deficiency is associated with insulin resistance, the metabolic syndrome and poor stress response. There is also evidence of an association between magnesium deficiency and pathological anxiety. Magnesium is important for stabilising blood pressure, so it is not surprising that high blood pressure is also symptomatic of inadequate intake.

The best sources of this mineral include nuts and leafy greens – which, of course are precisely what you will be eating in the evening as you follow *The Body Clock Diet*. Dark leafy greens such as spinach, broccoli, kale and cabbage have a very low carbohydrate content so are ideal in the evening. Nuts too are a rich source of magnesium, with very little carbohydrate (especially Brazils), so together they create a winning combination.

Being mindful

Even with these dietary changes, you still need to deal with the stress in your life. You may not be able to change your job, or your family, but you can change the way you react to stress. It's all about perception.

If you are suffering from prolonged stress you need to

find stress management techniques that suit you. Exercise must be part of that management, and you can read about stress and exercise later. Gentle, relaxing techniques may be more appropriate. Yoga for example is ideal because it combines relaxation and exercise. You may feel you need a talking therapy, in which case a professional stress therapist may be appropriate.

'Mindfulness' is currently enjoying great popularity, and with good reason. Mindfulness is a form of secular meditation, which promotes a focussed state of calm awareness and being 'in the moment'. Thoughts and feelings are observed without judgement or reaction. It is easier said than done, which is why classes have sprung up everywhere, offering guidance. Mindfulness is highly recommended as a stress management technique, and in overweight and obese individuals has been found to help normalise eating patterns.

Take your time

Taking time over your food - specifically, chewing each mouthful well, will not only aid relaxation, it will reduce your appetite and increase your sense of fullness. This effect has been observed in research, including one American study of 30 healthy women who reported greater satiety, and less desire to eat, when food was chewed for longer than usual. You might, quite reasonably, think that this effect was reported because the women knew they were being studied, and consequently their perception of satiety and appetite was altered. But the results of another study, examining gut hormones, suggest that the effects of chewing food thoroughly are not all in your mind – they are in your gut too. A group of men were found to not only eat less after chewing their food 40 times compared to a test group who chewed only 15 times, they were also found to have significantly reduced levels of the hormone ghrelin and increased levels of CCK. Ghrelin, you may recall, is produced in the stomach and tells the brain you are hungry. CCK is released from the small intestine and tells the brain when you've had enough. As the authors of the study state, improving chewing frequency could be a useful tool in the fight against obesity. Forty seems to be the magic number. Another study of pizza-guzzling men found that, compared with fifteen chews per mouthful, forty chews resulted in reduced hunger and preoccupation with food, reduced desire to eat, greater CCK and lower ghrelin levels. So as part of your relaxation programme, take the time to eat your food properly and mindfully, chewing each mouthful so thoroughly that you are able to distinguish more subtle, delicate flavours.

(23) Exercise right

The pain passes, but the beauty remains. (Pierre Auguste Renoir)

There's good news and there's bad news on the exercise front.

First, the bad news. Many of you may have already noticed that, despite claims and hopes to the contrary, exercise has little - if any - direct effect on weight. If you exercise without making appropriate dietary changes you can expect naff-all results. The good news is that exercise can have a significant indirect effect on weight. The trick is to exercise smart: do the right kind of exercise at the right time, and for the right reasons. Confused? Of course you are, so here's what you need to know about exercise and fat burning.

Your storage capacity

A major review of the research into the effect of exercise on weight loss – a total of 43 studies involving nearly 3,500 overweight or obese participants – found that those who carried out regular, high intensity exercise, without making any dietary changes, for between 3 and 12 months, enjoyed average weight loss of 1.5 kilos. That's right: all that exercise, for all that time, for a measly 1.5 kilos. The people involved in these studies didn't come away completely empty-handed - they did benefit from reduced blood pressure, which I'm sure was a comfort to them.

Perhaps the poor results experienced by regular exercisers are inevitable, because it is impossible to burn a lot of stored fat through exercise alone. The largest energy store in the human body is adipose tissue. A lean adult has in the region of 80,000 calories of potential energy squirrelled away as fat – enough to complete 25 marathon races. This supply is 40 times greater than the amount of energy stored as glycogen in muscles and the liver. And that's just a thin person. That, I'm afraid, is the brutal reality of human fat storage capacity. We're all potential big box warehouses.

On the plus side, when you combine exercise with the

right type of diet, you can expect to shrink that warehouse capacity to cupboard space. That is because of the *indirect* effect that exercise has on fat burning. There are three main ways that exercise will significantly supplement *The Body Clock Diet* and make it all happen faster and more efficiently.

Indirect effects

First, exercise improves insulin control, and the better your insulin control, the more you burn fat rather than store it. As you saw in part three, poorly controlled insulin plays a major role in increasing your fat stores. A sedentary lifestyle is known to reduce insulin sensitivity, but the more exercise you do, the more your body is able to respond to and control insulin. Combining exercise with a diet designed to optimise insulin control accelerates your fat burning capacity.

Second, exercise influences the secretion of two important hormones. It increases output of growth hormone, which as you saw in part five is important for burning fat at night. Exercise also helps normalise levels of the stress hormone cortisol. Cortisol mobilises energy, and levels are naturally high in the morning and fall towards evening, in preparation for sleep and the body's nocturnal metabolic activities. Intense exercise stimulates the production of cortisol, which may interfere with sleep. It therefore suits your body clock to carry out aerobic exercise earlier in the day, when cortisol levels are naturally higher. Ideally, make sure any intense exercise is carried out in the morning or early to mid afternoon.

Yoga, on the other hand, has been found to decrease cortisol levels, suggesting that gentle exercise is more appropriate in the evening. Evenings are for winding down and relaxing, and getting ready for some serious nocturnal fat burning.

Third, exercise helps maintain weight loss once it has been achieved – in fact it has been described as 'critical' for weight loss maintenance. Eating right will facilitate your weight loss, and exercise will keep it off. Research suggests that 60-90 minutes a day of moderate to intense physical activity is required to achieve this effect. That's quite a lot, but then, human beings are built to move. Sedentary lifestyles are alien to our genetic make-up; our genes were forged in an environment where everyday outdoor physical activity was the norm.

Slow, slow, quick quick slow

Fortunately you do not need to engage in weekly marathon runs or attain superhuman status to increase your metabolic rate. Running long distances has not been found to be more beneficial to health than walking long distances; rather, studies suggest that regular exercise and sustained movement with rest and recovery periods throughout the day are more effective than continuous activity. Modern hunter-gatherers habitually walk several miles a day, with intermittent bursts of high intensity activity, usually running. They also spend time digging, lifting and building.

There are lots of good reasons to engage in daily exercise. Exercise does all sorts of brilliant things. It keeps you fit and improves your health overall. It also makes you feel better – more energised, positive and uplifted. Ideally, you will exercise as much as possible outdoors, but if your work involves sitting for long periods (like me), move around as much as possible. I have a yoga mat by my desk and after an hour of work will get up and do about 10 minutes of stretching, or go outside and do some gardening. Most mornings I go for a slow jog for about thirty to forty minutes. A sedentary job means you have to be aware of your posture and the need to work your bones and muscles. Whatever you do for a living, you have to factor in time and space for physical activity throughout the day.

Takeaway

- A calorie-restricted diet can slow down thyroid hormone production and result in weight gain
- The metabolic syndrome can inhibit thyroid hormone
- Iodine is crucial for thyroid hormone production, but deficiency is a problem worldwide, including the UK
- Deficiency of zinc, iron and selenium can also cause thyroid insufficiency
- Certain goitrogenic foods should be avoided, but only if you have hypothyroidism and only if they are uncooked
- Stress can make you fat, by raising levels of the hormone cortisol and causing cravings
- The abdominal region is most responsive to cortisol
- Omega-3 fatty acids and magnesium help normalise cortisol output
- Mindfulness and yoga can help reduce stress
- Chewing your food properly reduces appetite and increases satiety
- Exercise has little direct effect on fat burning
- Exercise indirectly encourages fat burning by improving insulin sensitivity
- Exercise stimulates growth hormone and cortisol. Intense aerobic exercise is best avoided in the evening.
- Exercise helps maintain weight loss once it has been achieved

Part Seven

NOT THE END

 Stay successful

So here you are. You've lost the weight you set out to lose, and my guess is that once you got into your stride the process was much less restrictive than you anticipated. If you are someone with a history of dieting, of eating less and moving more, following *The Body Clock Diet* must have been a breeze by comparison.

You can continue eating this way for as long as you like; it's only natural. By doing so, you'll stay at your ideal weight. We spent hundreds of thousands of years evolving on this sort of diet, yet in the blink of an eye and the birth of an industry we have managed to demolish the relationship between our food and our genetic makeup. But now the true human diet has come home.

In terms of nutrition, you are not missing out on anything you need on this programme. Your thyroid and metabolism have been fortified, you have lost weight but also gained energy, improved your mood and concentration... what is it like to feel human again?

Think of *The Body Clock Diet* as a baseline to which you can return whenever you want. If on occasion you overdo things, you can relax in the knowledge that you can always return to base to avert any potential weight gain. The following table provides details of foods you can, within moderation, add to your programme every now and again. I've given some general guidance on frequency of consumption, but in practice it's down to you – you'll soon work out what you can and cannot get away with. Note that I have not included snacks in your maintenance programme. Snacking is a habit I strongly urge you to continue avoiding.

Whatever you do, do not lose sight of the fundamentals of the original human diet, the diet most suited to the human body, one that does not promote body fat or the sort of cravings that can lead to an unhealthy relationship with food.

Maintenance programme – foods which can be added to your daily diet

Food	Frequency	Notes
Porridge	Three times weekly max	Has a low GI if made with jumbo (as opposed to small) oats.
Honey	1-2 teaspoons with porridge or yogurt	Despite containing sugars, honey is a highly nutritious food. It also has high levels of antioxidants called polyphenols, which have remarkable medicinal properties.
Wholemeal bread	Two slices once or twice a week	Most breads have a high GI and bread generally is of no special nutritional value. If you love it, the healthiest type is probably traditional sourdough. Sourdough has a medium GI.
Yogurt – live (bio) and natural	Three times weekly max	Live yogurt can be a pleasant breakfast alternative. You can sweeten with your honey allowance and/or add fruit.
Milk and cream	Three times weekly max	So delicious (cream, anyway) it would be a shame not to.
Beans and lentils	Three times weekly max	Examples include adzuki, borlotti, black-eye, butter, haricot, chick pea, red kidney and black. Not including tinned baked beans. Nutritious, low GI carbohydrates with reasonable levels of protein.
Roots and tubers	Once or twice a week	Rather than potatoes, you could try the more nutritious sweet potato (no relation). Other starchy vegetables such as swede and turnips also offer decent nutrition.
Dried fruit	Once or twice a week	If you really fancy something sweet, dried fruit is your best option. Contains concentrated fructose, but some decent nutrients.
Higher carbohydrate fruits: apple, orange, grapes, mango, pear, cherries, pineapple	One portion daily	If you fancy a bit more variety, these options are highly nutritious and contain those all-important phytochemicals.

The Body Clock Diet

Appendix 1

FOOD TABLES

The following tables provide a guide to what to eat, and what not to eat, whilst following *The Body Clock Diet*, and a reminder of why.

What to eat

Fruit	
On the menu	**Details**
Berries (all types, inc. strawberries, raspberries, blueberries), plum, melon, kiwi, peach, satsuma, tangerine	Two pieces/portions daily, any time in the morning. Low carbohydrate content
Olives	Despite being a fruit they contain virtually no carbohydrate. May be eaten instead of nuts before dinner or as part of a meal

What not to eat

Fruit	
Off the menu	**Because**
Banana & plantain	High carbohydrate content
Apple, orange, grapes, mango, pear, cherries, pineapple	Medium to high carbohydrate content – stick with low carb fruits
Dried fruit	Concentrated fructose

What to eat

Vegetables

On the menu	Details
Steamed leafy greens: spinach, spring greens, Swiss chard, etc.	Especially important in the evening: high magnesium content, very low carbohydrate content
Brassicas: cabbage, cauliflower, kale, broccoli, bok choy	Especially important in the evening: high magnesium content, very low carbohydrate content
Salad leaves	Dress generously with extra virgin olive oil and any vinegar of your choice. Avoid raw watercress if you have a thyroid disorder
Peppers, aubergines	Low carbohydrate content
Peas (inc. mange tout & sugar snaps)	Unlike other legumes, they have a low carbohydrate content. Exception opposite:
Tomatoes, cucumber, marrow, courgette, pumpkin, squash ('fruit' vegetables)	All high water, low carbohydrate content
Green (string) beans, runner beans	Low carbohydrate content
Avocado	Technically a fruit but eat as a salad vegetable. Very little carbohydrate content
Misc. vegetables: asparagus, fennel, leaks, mushrooms, celery, chicory, carrots	Low to very low carbohydrate content

What not to eat

Vegetables and other plant foods

Off the menu	Because
Potatoes and other starchy tubers and roots*: sweet potatoes, yams, parsnips, celeriac, turnip/swede	High carbohydrate content
Sweetcorn	High carbohydrate content
Legumes – beans and lentils – chick peas, aduki, broad, butter, black-eye, haricot etc.	High carbohydrate content
Quinoa	High carbohydrate to protein ratio
Mushy peas	High carbohydrate content

* The exception being carrots which have a fairly low carbohydrate content

What to eat

Meat

On the menu	Details
Red meat: beef, lamb, pork, rabbit, venison	High protein, zinc, B12, iron
Processed meats: ham, sausages, bacon	These are fine in terms of weight loss. However – sausages should have a high meat content (at least 80%). Quality sausages do not usually contain preservatives. For health reasons, limit ham and bacon (contain preservatives).
Poultry: chicken, turkey, pheasant, duck, geese, guinea fowl, quail	High protein, zinc, B12

Fish

On the menu	Details
Oily fish: mackerel, trout, salmon, herring, white bait, sardines, pilchards, anchovies	High protein Rich dietary source of omega-3 fatty acids EPA and DHA Good source of B12, iodine and selenium Preferably wild, not farmed
White fish: plaice, sole, cod, coley, haddock, monkfish, hake, halibut, skate, whiting, pollack	High in protein. Most are good source of B12, iodine and selenium
Shellfish: crab, lobster, barnacles, prawns, crayfish, oysters, mussels, squid, octopus	Protein-rich. Also reasonable source of EPA and DHA. Rich in zinc. Good source of B12, iodine and selenium

What not to eat

Meat

Off the menu

Any type of meat coated in breadcrumbs

Because

High carbohydrate/refined omega-6 content

Fish

Off the menu

Any type of fish coated in breadcrumbs or batter

Because

High carbohydrate/refined omega-6 content

What to eat

Dairy

On the menu	Details
Cheese (with exceptions, opposite)	Whey is removed in the cheese making process. Source of protein
Butter	Almost entirely fat; no whey

Cooking fats and oils

On the menu	Details
Butter	Saturated fat – good for cooking
Lard	Saturated fat – good for cooking
Extra virgin olive oil	Monounsaturated fat - good for cooking and dressings. If it isn't extra virgin it has undergone the same refining processes as other cooking oils
Coconut oil	Saturated fat – good for cooking
Palm oil	Saturated fat. Sometimes found on ingredients list. You may prefer to source sustainable palm oil
Cold-pressed rape-seed oil	A (bland) alternative to EV olive oil; predominantly omega-3
Mayonnaise made with cold-pressed rapeseed oil	Available from larger supermarkets. Good alternative to other mayos that are high in omega-6

What not to eat

Dairy

Off the menu	Because
Milk	With the exception of most cheeses and butter, dairy contains the protein whey - causes insulin spikes
Yogurt	Contains whey
Ricotta and cottage cheese	Ricotta is made from whey. Cottage cheese contains some whey
Cream, inc. crème fraiche	Whey rich
Scandinavian 'brown' cheeses	Whey rich
Buttermilk	Whey rich

Cooking fats and oils

Off the menu	Because
Margarines and spreads, including spreadable butters	High carbohydrate/refined omega-6 content
Corn oil	High in refined omega-6. Check food in jars, tubs, tins etc. for this ingredient
Soya oil	High in refined omega-6. Check food in jars, tubs, tins etc. for this ingredient
Nut and seed cooking oils – sunflower, sesame, safflower, walnut	High in omega-6. Check food in jars, tubs, tins etc. for this ingredient. Cold-pressed oils – for example walnut or sesame - may occasionally be used as dressings, but never heated

What to eat

Other foods

On the menu	Details
Nuts: Brazils, cashews, hazelnuts, macadamias, almonds, pistachios, walnuts, pecans	Plain; not roasted in oil. A small handful half an hour or less before evening meal. May also form part of meal. Brazils are especially high in selenium and magnesium
Seeds: sunflower, pine-nuts, linseeds	May form part of meal
Eggs	Good protein
Edible seaweeds	Iodine-rich. Good in soups, stews, stir-fries

What to drink

On the menu	Details
Water	Still, fizzy or filtered
Tea	Preferably green (or white) tea but black tea also acceptable
Coffee	Avoid lattes and cappuccinos
Wine	In low to moderate quantities only. Preferably red – high in resveratrol

What not to eat

Other foods

Off the menu	Because
Cereal grains and their products: wheat, rice, corn, barley, rye etc.	High carbohydrate content. Low nutritional value
Added sugar in all its forms: glucose (dextrose) sucrose, fructose, lactose, maltose	Pure carbohydrate. No sweetener required
Honey	High in sugars

What not to drink

Off the menu	Because
Sugar-sweetened soft drinks	High carbohydrate content
Chemically sweetened soft drinks	No better than sugar-sweetened
Fruit juice	Concentrated fructose
Spirits	High alcohol content
Fortified wines (sherry, port etc.)	High carbohydrate content
Beers	Some beers have a very low carbohydrate content but there is variation between beers. Unless you are certain of the carbohydrate content, best avoided

Appendix 2

MEAL IDEAS

Breakfast ideas

- Two premium sausages and an egg with mushrooms and tomatoes. Grilled or fried in extra virgin olive oil/coconut oil
- Two slices of bacon, fried egg and a couple of slices of black pudding with mushrooms and tomatoes.
- Two large, hardboiled eggs, sliced. Topped with a few anchovy fillets and olives
- Two large hardboiled eggs, sliced, on a slice of ham or other cooked meat
- Three slices of cheddar cheese, topped with tomatoes. Handful of olives.
- Large tin (110g) of mackerel in brine (not oil, unless it is extra virgin olive oil) with olives and/or tomatoes
- Two large slices of ham or any cooked meat, such as roast pork, and a slice of cheese
- Large handful of mixed nuts with a large slice of Stilton cheese and a few olives
- Three small or two large slices of smoked salmon 'buttered' with cream cheese, sprinkled with dill. Sliced tomatoes.
- Two or three slices of smoked salmon, olives and tomatoes
- Scrambled eggs with smoked salmon and tomatoes
- Scrambled or poached eggs with a rasher of bacon, chopped.

- Cheese omelette with tomatoes and/or mushrooms
- Grilled kipper with mushrooms and tomatoes

Lunch/dinner ideas

- One large or two small pork chops
- One large or two small lamb chops
- Steak
- Roast chicken
- Three premium sausages
- Two fillets of smoked mackerel
- Cheese or bacon omelette
- Salmon fillet with prawns
- Whole mackerel or herring
- Chicken/pork/beef/seafood curry

Any of the above, with your choice of vegetables from appendix 1.

Suggested lunchbox items

Cold omelette with cheese, ham or bacon
Tuna & egg mash with mayonnaise (made with cold-pressed rapeseed oil)
Tinned salmon with mayonnaise (made with cold-pressed rapeseed oil)
Two smoked mackerel fillets
Large tin (110g) of mackerel
Cold wild salmon fillet with prawns
3-4 cold slices meat/ham
3 cooked (premium) sausages
Large portion of grated cheddar or other cheese
Mozzarella with avocado and tomato (*insalata tricolore*)
Prawns with avocado and mayo (made with cold-pressed rapeseed oil)
Chicken leg
Leftovers from the previous evening

With

Any two vegetables from the list in appendix one.
If you are having a salad, make a dressing with extra virgin olive oil and balsamic vinegar (or any other vinegar)

REFERENCES

INTRODUCTION

Bates, B. Lennox, A., Prentice, A., Bates, C. *et al* (2014). National Diet and Nutrition Survey Rolling Programme (NDNS RP). Results from years 1-4 (combined) (2008/09 - 2011/12). London, Food Standards Agency and Public Health England

Health & Social Care Information Centre (2015). *Statistics on Obesity, Physical Activity and Diet: England 2015.* National Statistics

PART ONE

(1)   Never count calories

Cannon, G. and Einzig, H. (1983). *Dieting Makes You Fat.* London: Century Publishing

Keys, A., Brozek. J., Henschel, A. *et al* (1950). *The Biology of Human Starvation*. Minnesota: University of Minnesota Press

Dulloo, A. G., Jacquet, J. and Montani, J. P. (2012). 'How dieting makes some fatter: from a perspective of human body composition autoregulation', *Proceedings of the Nutrition Society* 71(03): 379-389

Pietiläinen, K. H., Saarni, S. E., Kaprio, J. and Rissanen, A. (2012). 'Does dieting make you fat? A twin study', *International Journal of Obesity* 36(3): 456-464

National Health Service www.nhs.uk accessed March 2014

PART TWO

Cross, M. (2013) *Food and How to Make a Healthy Meal of it.* CrossWords

(2) Drink the right kind of tea

Westerterp-Plantenga, M. S., Lejeune, M. P. and Kovacs, E. M. (2005). 'Body weight loss and weight maintenance in relation to habitual caffeine intake and green tea supplementation', *Obesity Research* 13(7): 1195-1204

Hursel, R., Viechtbauer, W. and Westerterp-Plantenga, M. S. (2009). 'The effects of green tea on weight loss and weight maintenance: a meta-analysis', *International Journal of Obesity* 33(9): 956-961

(3) Get your coffee kicks

Ding, M., Bhupathiraju, S. N., Chen, M. *et al* (2014). 'Caffeinated and decaffeinated coffee consumption and risk of type 2 diabetes: A systematic review and a dose-response meta-analysis', *Diabetes Care* 37(2): 569-586

(4) Jettison the juicer

Seneff, S., Wainwright, G. and Mascitelli, L. (2011). 'Is the metabolic syndrome caused by a high fructose, and relatively low fat, low cholesterol diet', *Archives of Medical Science* 7(1): 8-20

Bray, G.A. (2007). 'How bad is fructose?', *American Journal of Clinical Nutrition* 86(4):895-896

Elliot, S.S., Keim, N.L., Stern, J.S. *et al* (2002). 'Fructose, weight gain and the insulin resistance syndrome', *American Journal of Clinical Nutrition* 76(5): 911-922

PART THREE

(5) Eat when you're ready

Hucklebridge, F. H., Clow, A., Abeyguneratne, T. *et al* (1999). 'The awakening cortisol response and blood glucose levels', *Life Sciences* 64(11): 931-937

Purslow, L.R., Sandhu, M.S., Forouhi, N. *et al* (2008). 'Energy intake at breakfast and weight change: prospective study of 6,764 middle-aged men and women', *American Journal of Epidemiology* 167(2): 188-192

(6) Control your insulin

Larsen, C.S. (2003). 'Animal source foods and human health during evolution', *Journal of Nutrition* 133(11): 3893S-3897S

Verginelli, F., Aru, F., Battista, P. and Mariani-Costantini, R. (2009) 'Nutrigenetics in the light of human evolution', *Journal of Nutrigenetics and Nutrigenomics*: 2:91-102
Cordain, L. (1999). 'Cereal grains: Humanity's double-edged sword', *World Review of Nutrition and Dietetics* 84:19-73ß

Armelagos, G.J. and Harper, K.N. (2005). 'Genomics at the origins of agriculture, part two', *Evolutionary Anthropology* 14:109-121

Steen, E., Terry, B.M., Rivera, E.J. *et al* (2005). 'Impaired insulin and insulin-like growth factor expression and signaling mechanisms in Alzheimer's disease – is this type 3 diabetes?', *Journal of Alzheimer's Disease* 7: 53-80

Sims-Robinson, C., Bhumsoo, K., Rosko, A. and Feldman, E.L. (2010). 'How does diabetes accelerate Alzheimer disease pathology?', *Nature Reviews Neurology* 6.10: 551-559

Yancy, W.S., Olsen, M.K., Guyton, J.R. *et al* (2004). 'A low-carbohydrate, ketogenic diet versus a low-fat diet to treat obesity and hyperlipidemia', *Annals of Internal Medicine* 140:769-777

Krieger, J.W., Sitren, H.S., Daniels, M.J. and Langkamp-Henken, B. (2006). 'Effects of variation in protein and carbohydrate intake on body mass and composition during energy restriction: a meta-regression', *American Journal of Clinical Nutrition* 83: 260-274

Westman, E.C., Feinman, R.D., Mavropoulos, J.C. *et al* (2007). 'Low-carbohydrate nutrition and metabolism', *American Journal of Clinical Nutrition* 86(2):276-284

Blom, W. A., Lluch, A., Stafleu, A. *et al* (2006). 'Effect of a high-protein breakfast on the postprandial ghrelin response', American Journal of Clinical Nutrition 83(2): 211-220

Purslow, L.R., Sandhu, M.S., Forouhi, N. *et al* (2008). 'Energy intake at breakfast and weight change: prospective study of 6,764 middle-aged men and women', *American Journal of Epidemiology* 167(2): 188-192

Leidy, H. J., Ortinau, L. C., Douglas, S. M., and Hoertel, H. A. (2013). 'Beneficial effects of a higher-protein breakfast on the appetitive, hormonal, and neural signals controlling energy intake regulation in overweight/obese, "breakfast-skipping," late-adolescent girls', *American Journal of Clinical Nutrition* 97(4): 677-688

(7) Don't go soft

Malik, V.S., Popkin, B.M., Bray, G.A. *et al* (2010). 'Sugar-sweetened beverages, obesity, type 2 diabetes mellitus and cardiovascular disease risk', *Circulation* 121: 1356-1364

Malik, V.S., Schulze, M.B. and Hu, F.B. (2006). 'Intake of sugar-sweetened beverages and weight gain: a systematic review', *American Journal of Clinical Nutrition* 84(2): 274-288

Ferland, A., Brassard, P. and Poirier, P. (2007). 'Is aspartame really safer in reducing the risk of hypoglycemia during exercise in patients with type 2 diabetes?', *Diabetes Care* 30(7): e59

Polyák, É., Gombos, K., Hajnal, B. et al (2010). 'Effects of artificial sweeteners on body weight, food and drink intake', *Acta Physiologica Hungarica* 97(4): 401-407

PART FOUR

(10)   Fan those fat-burning flames

Layman, D.K., Evans, E.M., Erickson, D. *et al* (2009). 'A moderate-protein diet produces sustained weight loss and long-term changes in body composition and blood lipids in obese adults', *Journal of Nutrition* 139(3): 514-521

Leidy, H. J., Mattes, R. D. and Campbell, W. W. (2007). 'Effects of acute and chronic protein intake on metabolism, appetite, and ghrelin during weight loss', *Obesity* 15(5): 1215-1225

Weigle, D. S., Breen, P. A., Matthys, C. C. *et al* (2005). 'A high-protein diet induces sustained reductions in appetite, ad libitum caloric intake, and body weight despite compensatory changes in diurnal plasma leptin and ghrelin concentrations', *American Journal of Clinical Nutrition* 82(1): 41-48

Johnstone, A. M., Horgan, G. W., Murison, S. D. *et al* (2008). 'Effects of a high-protein ketogenic diet on hunger, appetite, and weight loss in obese men feeding ad libitum', *American Journal of Clinical Nutrition* 87(1): 44-55

Druce, M. R., Wren, A. M., Park, A. J. *et al* (2005). 'Ghrelin increases food intake in obese as well as lean subjects', *International Journal of Obesity* 29(9): 1130-1136

Raybould, H. E. (2007). 'Mechanisms of CCK signaling from gut to brain', *Current Opinion in Pharmacology* 7(6): 570-574

Paddon-Jones, D., Westman, E., Mattes, R. D *et al* (2008). 'Protein, weight management, and satiety', *American Journal of Clinical Nutrition* 87(5): 1558S-1561S

Delzenne, N., Blundell, J., Brouns, F. *et al* (2010). 'Gastrointestinal targets of appetite regulation in humans', *Obesity Reviews* 11(3): 234-250

Seshadri, S., Beiser, A., Selhub, J. *et al* (2002). 'Plasma homocysteine as a risk factor for dementia and Alzheimer's disease', *New England Journal of Medicine* 346(7): 476-483

Schnyder, G., Roffi, M., Flammer, Y. (2002). 'Effect of homocysteine-lowering therapy with folic acid, vitamin B12, and vitamin B6 on clinical outcome after percutaneous coronary intervention. The Swiss Heart Study: a randomized controlled trial', *Journal of the American Medical Association* 288(8): 973-979

Martin, F.M., Armstrong, L.E. and Rodriguez, N.R. (2005). 'Dietary protein intake and renal function', *Nutrition and Metabolism*: 2:25

Bonjour, J-P. (2005). 'Dietary protein: An essential nutrient for bone health', *Journal of the American College of Nutrition* 24(S6): 526S-536S

Fenton, T.R., Tough, S.C., Lyon, A.W. *et al* (2011). 'Causal assessment of dietary acid load and bone disease: a systematic review & meta-analysis applying Hill's epidemiologic criteria for causality', *Nutrition Journal* 10: 41

References

Eaton, B.S., Konner, M.J. and Cordain, L. (2010). 'Diet-dependent acid load, Paleolithic nutrition, and evolutionary health promotion', *American Journal of Clinical Nutrition* 91:295-7

(11) Say no whey

Salehi, A., Gunnerud, U., Muhammed, S. J. *et al* (2012). 'The insulinogenic effect of whey protein is partially mediated by a direct effect of amino acids and GIP on beta-cells' *Nutr Metab (Lond)*, 9(1): 48

(13) Eat your greens (and reds, blues, yellows …)

González-Castejón, M. and Rodriguez-Casado, A. (2011). 'Dietary phytochemicals and their potential effects on obesity: a review', *Pharmacological Research* 64(5): 438-455

(14) Eat fat to burn fat

Samaha, F. F., Iqbal, N., Seshadri, P. *et al* (2003). 'A low-carbohydrate as compared with a low-fat diet in severe obesity', *New England Journal of Medicine* 348(21): 2074-2081

Ibrahim, M. M. (2010). 'Subcutaneous and visceral adipose tissue: structural and functional differences', *Obesity Reviews* 11(1): 11-18

Iyer, A., Fairlie, D. P., Prins, J. B. *et al* (2010). 'Inflammatory lipid mediators in adipocyte function and obesity', *Nature Reviews Endocrinology* 6(2): 71-82

Westman, E.C., Feinman, R.D., Mavropoulos, J.C. *et al* (2007). 'Low-carbohydrate nutrition and metabolism', *American Journal of Clinical Nutrition* 86(2):276-284

Sumithran, P., and Proietto, J. (2008). 'Ketogenic diets for weight loss: a review of their principles, safety and efficacy', *Obesity Research & Clinical Practice* 2(1): 1-13

Grieb, P., Kłapcinska, B., Smol, E., *et al* (2008). 'Long-term consumption of a carbohydrate-restricted diet does not induce deleterious metabolic effects', *Nutrition Research* 28(12): 825-833

(15) **Eat the right kind of fat**

Ailhaud, G., Massiera, F., Weill, P. *et al* (2006). 'Temporal changes in dietary fats: Role of n-6 polyunsaturated fatty acids in excessive adipose tissue development and relationship to obesity. *Progress in Lipid Research*: 45(3): 203-236

Muhlhausler, B. S. and Ailhaud, G. P. (2013). 'Omega-6 polyunsaturated fatty acids and the early origins of obesity', *Current Opinion in Endocrinology, Diabetes and Obesity* 20(1): 56-61

Nunes, E., Peixoto, F., Louro, T. *et al* (2007). 'Soybean oil treatment impairs glucose-stimulated insulin secretion and changes fatty acid composition of normal and diabetic islets', *Acta Diabetologica* 44(3): 121-130

Jen, K. C., Buison, A., Pellizzon, M. *et al* (2003). 'Differential effects of fatty acids and exercise on body weight regulation and metabolism in female Wistar rats', *Experimental Biology and Medicine* 228(7): 843-849

Berry, E. M. (2001). 'Are diets high in omega-6 polyunsaturated fatty acids unhealthy?' *European Heart Journal Supplements* 3(suppl D): D37-D41

Buckley, J. D. and Howe, P. R. (2010). 'Long-chain omega-3 polyunsaturated fatty acids may be beneficial for reducing obesity - a review', *Nutrients* 2(12): 1212-1230

References

Noreen, E. E., Sass, M. J., Crowe, M. L. *et al* (2010). 'Effects of supplemental fish oil on resting metabolic rate, body composition, and salivary cortisol in healthy adults', *Journal of the International Society of Sports Nutrition* 7(31): 10-1186

Ramel, A., Martinez, A., Kiely, M. *et al* (2008). 'Beneficial effects of long-chain n-3 fatty acids included in an energy-restricted diet on insulin resistance in overweight and obese European young adults', *Diabetologia* 51(7): 1261-1268

Volek, J.S., Phinney, S.D., Forsythe, S.E. *et al* (2009). 'Carbohydrate restriction has a more favorable impact on the metabolic syndrome than a low fat diet', *Lipids* 44: 297-309

Hite, A. H., Feinman, R. D., Guzman, G. E. *et al* (2010). 'In the face of contradictory evidence: Report of the Dietary Guidelines for Americans Committee', *Nutrition* 26(10): 915-924

FAO/WHO (2008). Joint FAO/WHO Expert Consultation on Fats and Fatty Acids in Human Nutrition (10 - 14 November 2008, WHO, Geneva). Interim Summary of Conclusions and Dietary Recommendations on Total Fat and Fatty Acids

Assunção, M.L., Ferreira, H.S., dos Santos, A.F. *et al* (2009). 'Effects of dietary coconut oil on the biochemical and anthropometric profiles of women presenting abdominal obesity', *Lipids* 44:593-601

St-Onge, M., Ross, R., Parsons, W.D. and Jones, P.J.H. (2003). 'Medium-chain triglycerides increase energy expenditure and decrease adiposity in overweight men', *Obesity Research* 11:395-402

St-Onge, M., and Jones, P.J.H. (2002). 'Physiological effects of medium-chain triglycerides: Potential agents in the prevention of obesity', *The Journal of Nutrition* 132(3): 329-332

Nagao, K. and Yanagita, T. (2010). 'Medium-chain fatty acids: Functional lipids for the prevention and treatment of the metabolic syndrome', *Pharmacological Research* 61:208-212

Garg, A. (1998). 'High-monounsaturated-fat diets for patients with diabetes mellitus: a meta-analysis', *American Journal of Clinical Nutrition* 67(3): 577S-582S

Paniagua, J. A., De La Sacristana, A. G., Romero, I. *et al* (2007). 'Monounsaturated fat–rich diet prevents central body fat distribution and decreases postprandial adiponectin expression induced by a carbohydrate-rich diet in insulin-resistant subjects', *Diabetes Care* 30(7): 1717-1723

(16) Sup up your soup

Clegg, M. E., Ranawana, V., Shafat, A., and Henry, C. J. (2012). 'Soups increase satiety through delayed gastric emptying yet increased glycaemic response', *European Journal of Clinical Nutrition* 67(1): 8-11

(17) Drink the right alcohol, in the right amount

Sayon-Orea, C., Martinez-Gonzalez, M. A. and Bes-Rastrollo, M. (2011). 'Alcohol consumption and body weight: a systematic review', *Nutrition Reviews* 69(8): 419-431

Djoussé, L., Arnett, D. K., Eckfeldt, J. H. *et al* (2004). 'Alcohol consumption and metabolic syndrome: does the type of beverage matter?', *Obesity Research* 12(9): 1375-1385

Alkerwi, A., Boutsen, M., Vaillant, M. *et al* (2009). 'Alcohol consumption and the prevalence of metabolic syndrome: a meta-analysis of observational studies', Atherosclerosis 204(2): 624-635

Szkudelska, K. and Szkudelski, T. (2010). 'Resveratrol, obesity and diabetes', *European Journal of Pharmacology* 635(1): 1-8

Smoliga, J. M., Baur, J. A. and Hausenblas, H. A. (2011). 'Resveratrol and health – a comprehensive review of human clinical trials', *Molecular Nutrition & Food Research* 55(8): 1129-1141

PART FIVE

(18) Sleep it off

Kohsaka, A., and Bass, J. (2007). 'A sense of time: how molecular clocks organize metabolism', *Trends in Endocrinology & Metabolism* 18(1): 4-11

Mattson, M. P. and Wan, R. (2005). 'Beneficial effects of intermittent fasting and caloric restriction on the cardiovascular and cerebrovascular systems', *The Journal of Nutritional Biochemistry* 16(3): 129-137

Azevedo, F. R. D., Ikeoka, D. and Caramelli, B. (2013). 'Effects of intermittent fasting on metabolism in men', *Revista da Associação Médica Brasileira* 59(2): 167-173

Karatsoreos, I. N., Bhagat, S., Bloss, E. *et al* (2011). 'Disruption of circadian clocks has ramifications for metabolism, brain, and behavior', *Proceedings of the National Academy of Sciences* 108(4): 1657-1662

Waterhouse, J., Minors, D., Atkinson, G and Benton, D. (1997) 'Chronobiology and meal times: internal and external factors', *British Journal of Nutrition* 77(S1):S29-S38

Marcheva, B., Ramsey, K. M., Peek, C. B. *et al* (2013). 'Circadian clocks and metabolism'. In *Circadian Clocks* (pp. 127-155). Springer Berlin Heidelberg

Roenneberg, T., Allebrandt, K.V., Merrow, M. and Vetter, C. (2012). 'Social jetlag and obesity', *Current Biology* 22(10): 939-943

Knutson, K. L., and Van Cauter, E. (2008). 'Associations between sleep loss and increased risk of obesity and diabetes', *Annals of the New York Academy of Sciences* 1129(1): 287-304

Sharma, S. and Kavuru, M. (2010). 'Sleep and metabolism: *An overview', International Journal of Endocrinology Article ID 270832*

Beccuti, G. and Pannain, S. (2011). 'Sleep and obesity', *Current Opinion in Clinical Nutrition and Metabolic Care* 14(4): 402

Lam, J., and Ip, M.S. (2010). 'Sleep and the metabolic syndrome', *Indian Journal of Medical Research* 131: (2)

Møller, N., and Jørgensen, J. O. L. (2009). 'Effects of growth hormone on glucose, lipid, and protein metabolism in human subjects', *Endocrine Reviews* 30(2): 152-177

Berryman, D. E., List, E. O., Sackmann-Sala, L. *et al* (2011). 'Growth hormone and adipose tissue: beyond the adipocyte', *Growth Hormone & IGF Research* 21(3): 113-123

Copinschi, G. (2004). 'Metabolic and endocrine effects of sleep deprivation', *Essential Psychopharmacology* 6(6): 341-347

Taheri, S., Lin, L., Austin, D. *et al* (2004). 'Short sleep duration is associated with reduced leptin, elevated ghrelin, and increased body mass index', *PLoS Medicine*: 1(3) e62

(19)   Don't be a night owl

Arble, D.M., Bass, J., Laposky, A.D. *et al* (2009). 'Circadian timing of food intake contributes to weight gain', *Obesity* 17: 2100-2102

Salgado-Delgado, R., Angeles-Castellanos, M., Saderi, N. *et al* (2010). 'Food intake during the normal activity phase prevents obesity and circadian desynchrony in a rat model of night work', *Endocrinology* 151(3): 1019-1029

Antunes, L. C., Levandovski, R., Dantas, G. *et al* (2010). 'Obesity and shift work: chronobiological aspects', *Nutrition Research Reviews* 23(01): 155-168

PART SIX

(20)   Check your thermostat

Michalaki, M. A., Vagenakis, A. G., Leonardou, A. S. *et al* (2006). 'Thyroid function in humans with morbid obesity', *Thyroid* 16(1): 73-78

Knudsen, N., Laurberg, P., Rasmussen, L. B. *et al* (2005). 'Small differences in thyroid function may be important for body mass index and the occurrence of obesity in the population', *Journal of Clinical Endocrinology & Metabolism* 90(7): 4019-4024

Ayturk, S., Gursoy, A., Kut, A. *et al* (2009). 'Metabolic syndrome and its components are associated with increased thyroid volume and nodule prevalence in a mild-to-moderate iodine-deficient area', *European Journal of Endocrinology* 161(4): 599-605

Volek, J.S., Sharman, M.J., Love, D.M. *et al* (2002) 'Body composition and hormonal responses to a carbohydrate-restricted diet', *Metabolism* 51(7): 864-870

Zimmermann, M. B., Jooste, P. L., and Pandav, C. S. (2008). 'Iodine-deficiency disorders', *The Lancet*: 372(9645): 1251-1262

Vitti, P., Rago, T., Aghini-Lombardi, F. and Pinchera, A. (2001). 'Iodine deficiency disorders in Europe', *Public Health Nutrition* 4(2b): 529-35

Zimmerman, M. and Delange, F. (2004). 'Iodine supplementation of pregnant women in Europe: a review of recommendations', *European Journal of Clinical Nutrition* 58: 979-84

Rayman, M., Sleeth, M., Walter, A and Taylor, A. (2008). 'Iodine deficiency in UK women of child-bearing age', *Proceedings of the Nutrition Society* 67(OCE8): E399

Vanderpump, M. P., Lazarus, J. H., Smyth, P. P. *et al* (2011). 'Iodine status of UK schoolgirls: a cross-sectional survey', *The Lancet*, 377(9782): 2007-2012

Rayman, M.P. (1997). 'Dietary selenium: Time to act', *British Medical Journal* 314: 387-388

Scientific Advisory Committee on Nutrition (2013). 'SACNE position statement on selenium and health.' SACN May 2013

Hess, S. Y., Zimmermann, M. B., Arnold *et al* (2002). 'Iron deficiency anemia reduces thyroid peroxidase activity in rats', *The Journal of Nutrition* 132(7): 1951-1955

Köhrle, J. (2005). 'Selenium and the control of thyroid hormone metabolism', *Thyroid* 15(8): 841-853

McDermott, M.T. and Ridgway, E.C. (2001). 'Subclinical hypothyroidism is mild thyroid failure and should be treated', *Journal of Clinical Endocrinology and Metabolism* 86(10): 4585-90

(21) **Cool your jets**

Epel, E. S., McEwen, B., Seeman, T. *et al* (2000). 'Stress and body shape: stress-induced cortisol secretion is consistently greater among women with central fat', *Psychosomatic Medicine* 62(5): 623-632

Tomiyama, A. J., Mann, T., Vinas, D. *et al* (2010). 'Low calorie dieting increases cortisol', *Psychosomatic Medicine* 72(4): 357-364

Kenny, P. J. (2011). 'Reward mechanisms in obesity: new insights and future directions', *Neuron* 69(4): 664-679

O'Connor, D.B., Jones, F., Connor, M. et al (2008). 'Effects of daily hassles and eating style on eating behavior', *Health Psychology* 27(1)(Suppl.): S20-S31

Dallman, M. F. (2010). 'Stress-induced obesity and the emotional nervous system', Trends in Endocrinology & Metabolism 21(3): 159-165

Adam, T. C., and Epel, E. S. (2007). 'Stress, eating and the reward system', *Physiology & Behavior* 91(4): 449-458

Delarue, J. O. C. P. R. L., Matzinger, O., Binnert, C., *et al* (2003). 'Fish oil prevents the adrenal activation elicited by mental stress in healthy men', *Diabetes & Metabolism* 29(3): 289-295

Rayssiguier, Y., Libako, P., Nowacki, W. and Rock, E. (2010). 'Magnesium deficiency and metabolic syndrome: stress and inflammation may reflect calcium activation', *Magnesium Research* 23(2): 73-80

Sartori, S. B., Whittle, N., Hetzenauer, A. and Singewald, N. (2012). 'Magnesium deficiency induces anxiety and

HPA axis dysregulation: modulation by therapeutic drug treatment', Neuropharmacology 62(1): 304-312

Daubenmier, J., Kristeller, J., Hecht, F. M. *et al* (2011). 'Mindfulness intervention for stress eating to reduce cortisol and abdominal fat among overweight and obese women: An exploratory randomized controlled study', *Journal of Obesity* 2011

(22) Take your time

Andrade, A. M., Greene, G. W. and Melanson, K. J. (2008). 'Eating slowly led to decreases in energy intake within meals in healthy women', *Journal of the American Dietetic Association* 108(7): 1186-1191

Li, J., Zhang, N., Hu, L. *et al* (2011). 'Improvement in chewing activity reduces energy intake in one meal and modulates plasma gut hormone concentrations in obese and lean young Chinese men', *American Journal of Clinical Nutrition* 94(3): 709-716

Zhu, Y., Hsu, W. H. and Hollis, J. H. (2013). 'Increasing the number of masticatory cycles is associated with reduced appetite and altered postprandial plasma concentrations of gut hormones, insulin and glucose', *British Journal of Nutrition* 110(02): 384-390

(23) Exercise right

Shaw, K., Gennat, H., O'Rourke, P. and Del Mar, C. (2006). 'Exercise for overweight or obesity', *Cochrane Database of Systematic Reviews* (4), Art No. CD003817

Horowitz, J. F. (2003). 'Fatty acid mobilization from adipose tissue during exercise', *Trends in Endocrinology & Metabolism* 14(8): 386-392

Houmard, J. A., Tanner, C. J., Slentz, C. A. *et al* (2004)

References

'Effect of the volume and intensity of exercise training on insulin sensitivity', *Journal of Applied Physiology* 96(1): 101-106

Mastorakos, G., Pavlatou, M., Diamanti-Kandarakis, E. and Chrousos, G. P. (2005). 'Exercise and the stress system', *Hormones* (Athens) 4(2): 73-89

West, J., Otte, C., Geher, K. *et al* (2004). 'Effects of Hatha yoga and African dance on perceived stress, affect, and salivary cortisol, *Annals of Behavioral Medicine* 28(2): 114-118

Hill, J. O. and Wyatt, H. R. (2005). 'Role of physical activity in preventing and treating obesity', *Journal of Applied Physiology* 99(2): 765-770

McGuigan, M. R., Egan, A. D. and Foster, C. (2004). 'Salivary cortisol responses and perceived exertion during high intensity and low intensity bouts of resistance exercise', *Journal of Sports Science and Medicine* 3: 8-15

Notes

Notes

Notes

Notes